# A Novel Approach to Everyday Life:

# "Get Lost, Girlfriend!"

BY
## SHARON
## LIVINGSTON, PH. D.

A Novel Approach to Everyday Life:
"Get Lost, Girlfriend!"
Copyright © 2016 Sharon Livingston, Ph. D.

Published by Psy Tech Inc.

Interior layout by Eileen Wiedbrauk of
eileenwiedbrauk.com

ISBN: 0692644156
ISBN-13: 978-0692644157

Also available as an ebook.

# A Novel Approach
## to Everyday Life:

## "Get Lost, Girlfriend!"

# PART ONE

BFN
My Best Friend For Never

# CHAPTER ONE:
## "Fruit Cake"

Arghhhh!!!! What is wrong with me! I just can't find any words. I want to scream. Sooooo frustrating.

Heavy sigh.

My lower back strains as I push myself up from my stability ball—my "chair" to my home office desk. My heavy lidded eyes survey my open concept living room, dining room, kitchen watching for sleeping Stewie, my sweet Shih Tzu, who I might stumble over. He likes to lounge on the parts of the rug that match his fluffy white and tan coat and I've been known to trip over him. My mind is distracted, again, as I walk over to the stainless steel side-by-side, double-door refrigerator.

I know a lot about refrigerators and how people feel about them from the research I did for Whirlpool a few years ago. Was so glad the house we bought had one that tested well with consumers. It was an indication that we had made the right choice with this house.

I pull open the door and stare. Hmmmph. Same stuff as half an hour ago. Nothing I feel like eating . . . or drinking. Green vegetables and Kombucha—a probiotic rich bubbly beverage—and some extra hard organic tofu. I close the door.

I walk around the island counter. And again. And again. Pace back and forth, pretend I'm exercising a little adding steps to the fit bit which resides on my bra strap ever tracking my every move. I open the sliding door to the deck, and carefully step out avoiding the slick ice patches. I remember that normally sure-footed Stewie slipped and pulled a muscle last week so I'd better be careful.

The shock of the chill feels good at first but then a shiver grips me and I come back inside.

I thought the cold air might wake me up, spark an idea. But, nooooo. Just jolts my senses a bit, but does nothing for my creativity or inspiration. I take a deep breath, exhale deeply feeling my body collapse into itself and slump into a chair at the dining room table as I stare through the wall that sports the artistic photographic close up of ice covered bare branches into the nowhere that exists beyond it.

I've been working hard on a book I want to publish. Well, I don't know how I can say I've been working hard when no words have escaped my mind, finger tips or key board in the past week. I think about what I want to say and then my mind wanders off into a myriad of directions as if it's trying to find a path to somewhere else.

My book. Right! My book. Uhmmm.

Come on Sharon, focus!

OK, ok. My book is about how we buy things. We all think we're so rational and logical but the truth is we make gut decisions and then find practical reasons to justify our desires.

For example, I love my Mac. Why? Well I might tell someone else who wanted to know why I switched that it's because it avoids viruses better than PC's; they have great customer support; they're user friendly and come with lots of built in apps; they work well with the iPhone and iPad—seamlessly . . . etc.

However, if I were true to myself and revealed my REAL feelings, it would be because I think it's cool to be a Mac user. Mac people are the artists of the world, soooo creative. AND I love the idea of being a creative person. You should see my Mac Book Pro "skin." It's a beautiful multicolor abstract in my favorite combination of reds, pinks, purples and touches of blue and green with tiny accents of yellow and orange that seem to swirl when you look at them, to ebb and flow like a yummy sea of edible paint. Everyone comments on it.

Or, another example.

I used to drive a Mercedes. Why? Because it was so well engineered, right? Well . . . maybe because I wanted to show I had arrived? Now I drive a cool burgundy Honda Accord that actually has better performance stats than my Mercedes did, but for 1/3 the price.

Not everyone will admit these underlying drivers. They don't realize them or want to acknowledge them if you ask them directly. They are afraid of revealing their true motivators for fear of looking strange, selfish, etc.

But me?

I'm a therapist and a consumer researcher with a Ph. D in psychology. I've actually interviewed over 62,000 people and I have tons of material. I've written many articles and been interviewed on radio, TV and many podcasts.

Yet here I sit, stuck, glued to my chair . . . my ball actually. Days on end. Just like this. Mind wandering. Antsy. Get up, walk around. Check to see if that sound was someone at the door, or maybe Gunner, the black lab pup from next door is on my deck again—he likes to visit old Zach and has been known to follow him in through the doggie door to stealthily raid his food bowl.

I try to change the scene by getting up to offer myself a different perspective—looking outback or opening the front door to see what if anything is going on with the neighbors. Or, I go sit in the bathroom and pick up a magazine that might inspire me.

Yayyy! An idea pops into my mind. I feel it. I think I'm on a roll, following an impulse, a glimmer of an idea. I run to the computer and as soon as I sit down—Poof—Uhm, what was it? Where did it go? I search my memory banks, mind's eyes roving back and forth looking but I'm empty, at a loss for words.

I softly touch the keys momentarily enjoying the sound of the clicks that remind me of a chorus line of girls tap dancing, hoping the action will stimulate thought, just taps no words. Mind once again drifting. I crack a silent joke for a little self amusement. "I used to be Snow White, but I drifted."

It's so hard to just sit there but there's nothing else I must do but write.

I again find meaningful ways to procrastinate:

- I check my email
- I think of a client or friend I should be calling
- I decide to exercise
- I give the pups quality play time
- I go food shopping
- I look something up that I've been meaning to pursue
- I decide to close my eyes for just a couple of minutes for a catnap and sleep like a dog

You know what I mean, I'm sure.

Haven't we all dragged our feet like this at various times.

[Another heavy sigh . . . .]

It reminds me of another time, a number of years ago when I was writing my mini dissertation for my Masters. [Little did I know then that it would be child's play compared to the real one to come a few years later. This was just a narrative not a full blown research project.]

I had gotten to a point where I had the same types of symptoms and distractions I was experiencing here and now—although at that time the critters were two adorable kitties, Sami and Nielsen, named after 2 marketing research agencies . . . [I take my work home.]

I would sit in front of the keyboard at a stalemate.

I had a deadline in order to get my degree.

I HAD to finish!

But, ugh, no words were coming. I just sat there twirling a strand of hair, around and around.

And, then as my thoughts wandered, I started feeling over an old hurt with my Dad. We had never been close. He was always angry at me for something. It felt like I was the bane of his existence. He only had eyes for my mom and my little sister. He loved my brother Jason. THEY could do no wrong.

But me? I was always at risk of being in trouble, getting his blast of cold fury; being frozen by fear of the angry hand that could catapult out of nowhere and

6

make painful contact with a body part. I mean, it's not as bad as I'm making it sound. He only actually beat me a few times that I can remember, but the fear of both actual pain and more importantly, the soul withering humiliation attached to the judgment, were always present when Dad was "in a mood." He never physically hit me after I was 9, but the threat was ever present and the contempt on his face was at least as harmful.

And where was my loving mother at these times?

Disappearing into the kitchen, cleaning up the mess of feeding the five us, as if, this was just a normal part of family life and she couldn't or wouldn't stop him from sullying my self-worth . . . so at least she could distract herself taking care of the kitchen.

After I graduated college and was on my own living and working in New York, and after several years of therapy, I went down to visit my folks in South Jersey. My parents were caterers and when they semi-retired they continued to maintain 2 kitchens in their home. On this particular day, the visit to my folks day, my father was working in the lower level kitchen. He called up to me to come help him. He was making a fruit cake.

['A fruit cake, really?' I hear myself thinking. 'We're Jewish, Dad. We don't eat fruitcake. But, Okayyy . . . whatever. You are kind of a fruit cake, so it's apropos I guess. I giggled to myself. I have to say that I really do enjoy my own jokes. And, I take after you right? Mom always said I was just like you and God knows I'm definitely a fruit cake in my own rights.']

So as I mentioned before, my father had his moods. I was always a little nervous with Dad because he could fly off the handle and do something weird when he was pissed off, like—scream, throw glass soda bottles, smash cartons of eggs, rip the phone out of the wall like he was eviscerating a fish, and TEAR UP my art work that I worked on for an entire college semester!!! Yeah, he did that. I shake my head at the memory.

When he wasn't having a temper tantrum, he tended to be quiet and not say much—just go about his business at work. He'd take out his aggression on a side of beef that he converted to various types of steaks and other cuts of meat to sell in the store. He'd hack away at the skinned flesh with deliberate whacks that were scary to watch. I generally used that time to go refresh the inventory on the shelves. There was always something that needed to be added or at least straightened out. But I could hear the pounding. When he was finished he'd take a big brush with metal bristles in both hands and scour the butcher block until all the blood was scraped off. But there was always a slightly oily residue left that was supposed to preserve the wood until the next massacre.

At home, he'd sit at the table, waiting to be served, staring into space, unblinking. When I was very little I used to wonder if being able to stare like that was something you were able to do when you became an adult. I also wondered, if when I was an adult I would grow to like peppermint instead of spearmint, lemon instead of cherry, chocolate ice cream instead of vanilla and any kind of sardines. The adults in my family seemed to like them. So it must be a function of age, right? Answer? None of the above . . . .

But, back to the fruit cake.

My father asked me to measure out some ingredients and put them into the big stainless steel bowl for him. I dutifully found the containers and meted out what I heard him say—what I was virtually, well . . . 99.44% CERTAIN he had said.

He turned and inspected the table. After scrutinizing how I had carried out his orders, his face began to color and glow as he exploded in rage.

He screamed into my face, spittle flying, called me some variation of stupid idiot—which in my family was worse than the worst F curse you can imagine—said I ruined it, I ruined something again, I ruined everything didn't I, because I never listened and I was so careless.

What was the matter with me?!

Why did he bother with me?!

Now he'd have to start all over again. Expletive, expletive . . . .

Imagine my dropped jaw, wide-eyed-stare of shock.

"But, but, that's what you said," I stammered meekly, my mouth suddenly parched, unable to swallow.

He kept yelling and hurling escalating insults.

And, then, I saw a knife on the oversized butcher block table.

I'm a highly visual person with an active imagination. As if someone else had taken control of me, I was brusquely projected into a terrifying reverie where I saw myself taking the knife and after only a second of hesitation plunging it into his back.

Now, I'm silently screaming inside, horrified that I was capable of such a violent thought . . . addressed at my own father!

I ran upstairs and hid in a bedroom too stunned and hurt to cry.

I fumbled for my cell and called Isabel, my therapist. I told her what happened and pleaded with her to take away the terrifying feeling and shame that I could be that angry, that murderous; I could actually see myself stabbing my father.

We went through the whole feeling discussion:

- It's important to distinguish thoughts vs. actions, she reminded me.
- Right, right, I know that.
- I thought about it, I didn't do it.
- I resisted taking the knife even though I was madly incensed.

- It's human to have feelings, human to think and feel anything/everything.
- People don't go to jail for thoughts and feelings.
- It's the action that counts.

I spoke to myself even as Isabel did. We both addressed me with calming understanding to cool me down—she out loud, me in my mind.

- You were angry.
- Who wouldn't be after being treated like that for YEARS.
- You did the right thing, leaving the lower level and calling for help as a way to take a breath and take care of yourself.
- You're ok.
- It's just a very angry feeling.

She had me talk some more, invited a few tears to wash out of my eyes, and after a while and a number of deep breaths, and me making a couple of very stupid, 5 year old jokes that brought forth her raucous signature laugh, I calmed down.

Even though I felt back in control, I couldn't bare being there anymore so I packed up my few things, made my goodbyes to my mother's tearful eyes [she always cried when any of us left] and drove back to New York.

This memory and others of his erratic explosions, being screeched at, struck, hit with a belt on my bare butt, humiliated and shamed; glared at with contempt; watching him lovingly play with my little sis while simultaneously remembering to turn and sneer at me, were going through my mind that day as I sat frozen in front of the keyboard trying to finish my Master's paper. I just didn't understand it.

Why? I shook my head back and forth. Why?

So, I took a short sabbatical from my report and wrote a letter to my father which respectfully expressed my sadness about our relationship. I no longer have the letter because I wrote it in long hand and mailed it to him. The one sentence I remember in particular was telling him I wanted to be one of the flowers in his well-tended garden.

Every spring he delighted in pruning, planting, watering, feeding, and growing the multitude of colorful flowers in the back yard of the home we lived in from the years I was 9-13. We moved a lot. But, when I think of where I grew up, that's the house I most often find myself migrating to as the one that represented home.

After living in a city with concrete and sidewalks and honking horns right outside the front door, walking out into an acre of fragrant flowers and sounds of birds singing in our backyard felt magical. There were four fruit trees along with the roses and lilacs and peonies—

two giant apple trees, a pear and a sour cherry. It was a fertile environment. Maybe Dad was happier there? I was no longer being hit, so maybe I was?

When my father read the letter, he called and told me he was coming to see me. He drove up to the house in northern New Jersey I was renting with a roommate. It was the old farmhouse on one acre of the 170 of the property. He was by himself [which was astounding in itself because he and Mom were inseparable] and for the one and only time in my life, sat with me on the enclosed back porch, where we drank tea and talked from our hearts. He stayed for an hour and left.

I was so touched and a little healed . . . AND, amazingly, I was able to go back to my assignment and finish my paper. My Master's advisor told me it was the best paper he had seen that year and while I got it in under the wire, it was worth the wait. Phewwww.

# CHAPTER TWO
## "The Year of the Horse"

This is the year of the horse, a time for many good things, I heard. Hmmmmm.

I don't know, because the first few months of this year, I've heard so many people talking about loss and bereavement among the coaches in our certification program. There are lots of people, so I get to hear lots of stories and honestly it hasn't been the easiest year in this regard for many people.

It got me to thinking. There are many types of losses we have to deal with on a daily basis—some big, some less consequential; some we take in stride, while others cut to the quick with profound effects. I think my procrastination at this time may have to do with a need to express my feelings about recent little and not so little losses and what they represent.

So taking a lesson from younger me, I'd like to tell you about my own personal journey over the last few months. Maybe it will help me get over my procrastination . . . .

## My "Personal Coffee Shop"

We had a cute little local coffee shop and luncheon place that catered very personally to its dwindling loyal base. Poor Sean tried sooooo hard, but he was a cook, not a marketer. ["Damn it Jim, I'm a doctor not a magician!" Sorry for the drift. I'm an avid Sci Fi Fan and love reruns of Star Trek.]

"Joe's Real Food" needed sprucing up AND air conditioning. Sean bought the place from Joe and kept the name to avoid confusing people. The food was great, the service was great, but people were going down the street to a cuter, cleaner, more comfortable café. Sean gave up after a year and a half of consistently losing money and closed on January 1st. It was soooo sad.

For 9 years, I had a happy ritual of getting up every morning, driving a couple of miles to see the people at Joe's, get some tea and a raw burger with raw broccoli that Sean made every morning for Stewie my Shih Tzu. Stewie has a very delicate tummy and has to eat raw. Sean accommodated, making my life a little easier . . . Before he closed, he taught me how to make the burger with a Hellmann's mayonnaise lid. Kind of cool, actually!

After Joe's locked its doors, I drove by the empty store every morning feeling sad and lost. Joe's was a daily touchstone that was a very comfortable and welcoming start to my morning.

I remember the day my mother passed. I walked into Joe's, saw Shelley and blurted out, "My mother died today."

She came around the counter, said "Awe honey, I'm so sorry," gave me a hug and we quietly stood there together for a moment. She was always reassuring to see every day, and particularly so, during that sad time.

After January 1st, I would go to Dunkin Donuts, get a decaf and head over to the parking lot of Market Basket with big and little dogs in the car, drink my warm drink and listen to a book on my iPhone, getting ready to exercise, and start work.

It just wasn't the same without the warm greetings from the people who opened Joe's and the other familiar faces that stopped for coffee at 6 am. Sometimes now, I'll run into someone who looks familiar but I don't really know them. If I think for a minute, I realize I know them from the take out counter at Joe's.

Things change—sometimes without our being ready to change along with them.

## My Ring

Two months ago, February, I decided that I had to get rid of the ice mass that had formed outside of the sliding doors to my deck. Stewie's little legs kept slipping every time he went out and I feared he'd pull his muscles. He came in one day with a limp, ugh. Being his 'mother,' I had to be responsible and protect him from further harm.

This was no small task. The ice was solid, hard and thick and blue and refused to respond to any kind of shovel. So I retrieved a hammer from our basement tool box, walked back upstairs through the foyer, through the kitchen, opened the sliding doors to the deck, deliberately yet cautiously stepped out and started striking that sucker with all my might.

Picture this—arms drawn up over head, holding the hammer with both hands, coming down as hard as I could—Thwok, thwok, thwok, thwok! Take that for hurting my sweet little Shih Tzu! Major THWOKK!!! It started cracking!! Yay! Success!!!!. More thwokking. It started to shatter. I kept at it, then I would sweep away the shards, sending them flying to the yard below—sweep left, sweep right, sweep back. Thwok, thwok, crunch, again. Soooo satisfying.

I continued thwokking and sweeping, and sweating even though it was frigid outside, until the deck was clear.

A while later I relaxed in a nice warm soothing tub with some fragrant essential oils; smelled so nice; so refreshing. As I got out of the tub, my eye caught my engagement ring to see that my diamond of 26 years was no longer in its setting.

Total shock. I stood frozen in time. [Well, I might have been better served and warmer with a towel but . . . ]

AHHHHH! A silent scream escaped my mouth.

How? Whah? It was so romantic when Glenn had given it to me? Where? Oh My God, Oh My God. I threw on a robe and searched the house. It must be here somewhere. Nooooo!

Oh My God . . . Did I lose it while hammering the ice?!! How will I ever find it?!

Long story short . . . It's gone. Such sadness . . . . Glenn was very sweet about it, but it felt sooooo wrong. Even a replacement wouldn't be the same thing. Maybe I'll find it in the grass, rocks, dirt that surround the deck . . . Maybe.

But, probably not.

## My Tooth

This is a very long story, so I'm just going to tell the end—Upper back tooth that had problems; went for deep laser therapy followed by antibiotics. Therapy failed, actually loosened the tooth and caused more infection—had to have it extracted and more antibiotics. This led to unpleasant, intense reactions to the long antibiotic treatment. That's just wrong; nauseous for three weeks, which meant the antibiotics had caused candida. Ugh. Now I have to treat that!

## My Mole

The day after my first oral surgery I went for a facial treatment. I see a doctor/aesthetician who does cool stuff for skin. As she was doing a light laser exfoliation of my face, she pointed out the little mole on my neck [that has been there for a lonngggg time—I was surprised that she was just seeing it] "Have you checked this with a Dermatologist. It looks like it could be Melanoma."

WHAAAAAT?! I thought? You drop the M word so casually? I've had this forever . . . holding my hysteria, I asked as calmly as I could, "Why do you think that?" She said, "Well it looks like it's changed? Do you check it every day? See this tiny black line?"

My heart is pounding. Melanoma? On my neck? Right under my chin? How much would they have to remove? Holy crap?! I looked to see if I could tell how serious she was.

She was serious.

Freaking out inside, heart palpitating, I hope I held it together on the outside, leaving as calmly as I could. It was Saturday. The dermatologist's office was closed for the weekend. All derms were closed, not just the one I had confidence in. Left an urgent message. Spent a very anxious weekend. They called me early, early Monday AM and got me in for a checkup by 10.

He scraped off the mole, said that to him it looked like an "AGE SPOT" that had thickened and sent it off for a biopsy. I said to him, "Really? Is that the technical name or do you just want to call me OLD!?" Ha ha ha ha. Not nice Doc. Don't you know what a big deal loss of youth is to us ladies?

I mean, don't physicians get some psychological training!?! I know the answer. It's no. Nor do they get any training on nutrition or natural approaches to health.

So I lost the mole, but didn't lose any years. Well I did lose a week of sanity worrying about the possible results. AND, he was right. It was an age spot. Long deep breath as I vow never to go back to the woman doctor who scared the living daylights out of me.

Hmmmm, maybe I should offer a light duty training program to physicians on bedside manner and the impact on patient loyalty. Hmmmm. Food for thought. Interesting idea.

# CHAPTER THREE
## "The Jill"

### My Friend

At the same time as the café, the ring, the tooth and the mole, my fabulous friend of all times who I couldn't believe I was so lucky to find . . . dumped me.

Was it because she was put off by my woes with my ring, tooth and mole? I don't think so. I actually never got a chance to tell her.

Two months ago I would have told you that I had a best friend. What a happy situation—a fantastic husband AND a wonderful female friend; 2 adorable dogs, a nice home in NH, great inspiring work with wonderful people who were on a mission to grow and help others. Just about close to perfect. [I mean, you know, it might have been nice to lose 5 lbs., get rid of a couple of wrinkles, sleep a little longer . . . but all in all, pretty great.]

My friend. [Let's call her Jill—Why Jill, you ask? Why not. And I like the name, wanted to be called Jill myself and she felt like a part of me. Hence, Jill.]

Jill and I met about 5 years ago when she came for treatment with the cranial sacral specialist who rented space in my office. I happened to be near the door when she walked in the first time. It was a moment frozen in time. Our eyes caught and widened. It was as if we had this sense of instant recognition with each other.

[According to Organizational Anthropologist, Judith Glazer, author of Conversational Intelligence—"Every conversation has an impact that takes place inside of us at the speed of .07 seconds. It registers at the cellular level."]

At that precise instant, both of our eyes lit up. We were drawn to each other, like mystical shimmery gossamer threads of some magnetically strong substance, connecting us, pulling us together. Something inside me shifted for that brief moment, time slowed and became luminously light and hard-to-move-heavy simultaneously. It was tough to pull away, to avert my eyes from hers.

But reality snapped like a taut rubber band shocking me back into real time. She was ascending the stairs to see Meryl and I had to get on a client call. We smiled broadly, murmured platitudes—nice to meet you—felt the tug, pulled away to go on and that was that.

I thought about it for a couple of seconds, mentally shrugged and went back to work.

Over the next couple of years, we continued to meet accidentally at different places in town—coffee shop, Barnes & Noble, supermarket, yoga studio, doctor's office . . . You might say, no big deal, small town—but I don't run into people like that. Just doesn't happen unless I intentionally go someplace to see someone. Isn't it true, you could live across the street from someone for years and never see them? I NEVER see Mike and Cheryl Biscayne who live cattycorner to us, but I was frequently running into Jill.

Then a couple of years ago, we both independently signed up for a weekend women's workshop that was held in the New Hampshire North Country. After a huge eyed "Hiiiiiii! we went into our separate parts of the meeting room. But then we kept gravitating to each other, working in the same circles on various exercises, laughing together, sitting at the same tables at lunch and dinner. We decided that the universe must have wanted us to pursue this relationship, because we were continually being thrown together. So before we left we made plans to visit at a local coffee shop in the next couple of weeks.

It was such fun to get to know her. She's smart, sensitive, and introspective; kind of crunchy granola

23

health conscious . . . We both awoke super early enjoying seeing the sunrise. She has two adorable girls, at that time 7 and 9. When I met them for the first time, she told me the older one looked at me, then back to her Mom, at me again and whispered to her in an awe filled voice, "Mommy, maybe she's the one!!"

The one? When Jill said that my heart sparked and started beating faster. The one? What did she mean? I wasn't sure but it felt special, I felt a little taller and excited to think that maybe I had found a friend after a long draught with no time to pursue and no close girl friend—just lots of casual acquaintances that were nice, but not very fulfilling.

We often met at that coffee shop. Sometimes, I'd bring my computer and work on a project. Sometimes she'd bring a book and read. We always ended up giggling over something, even if we first shared something uncomfortable, painful, frustrating, scary or sad. We had identical senses of humor and could easily send each other into peals of laughter. We could seemingly talk about whatever and clear it up enough to get back to our cheerful selves, restored by the total acceptance of each others' thoughts and feelings in our easy friendship. I felt so lucky. I hadn't felt so connected to another woman, hadn't had a "best" friend in many years.

It seemed like we were emotionally and intuitively twinned and entwined. We were in the same moods at the same time. If Jill was in a good mood, so was I. If everything seemed to be going wrong with one of us, the other was struggling that day too. We'd be amazed.

S—"How are you feeling?"

J—"Oh, I dunno, woke up feeling a little weird, like something was wrong, did you ever feel like that?"

S—"YES! That's exactly how I felt when I got up this morning!"

J—"Mercury must be in retrograde . . ."

S—"Or Uranus [pronounced your anus] is in retrograde . . ."

We'd both crack up, try to figure out what might be going on, but it was lighter now and really didn't matter that much.

It was intense. How could we both be feeling and dealing with the same stuff all the time?! It was strange but kind of comforting too. And, whenever we discussed what was up, we always felt better.

We quickly got into a habit of texting daily and talking a couple of times per week. I found myself checking my messages frequently looking for an indicator that there was a text from her.

Now it gets a little icky . . . Every now and then a day would go by without a word from her [although that was infrequent because I'd start the day out with a message, "Good Morning, Beauty!" And, she'd get back to me. Something newsy about a kid, the husband, the cat, the dog and we'd go about our day.]

I TRIED to temper my desire to text every morning before I heard from her, to make sure she would text first at least some of the time. You know, so it wouldn't seem like I wanted her more than she wanted me.

. . . Uh, oh! Sign of maybe something a little OCD? Addiction? Too involved? On those non-communicative days I'd later learn that she was depressed and retreated. I asked her if she wanted me to come after her at those times or if she preferred to be left alone. She said, "NOOO, please come after me. You always pull me out of it!"

So, I did. Rescuer me. Stupid me.

AND, we had long discussions about family, history, previous friends, current friends, coaching—because of course she's a coach—health and wellness, nutrition, exercise, psychology, impact of her being a mother vs. me being a career aunt. We had soooooo much in common.

Really, Sharon? You've never had kids. Career Aunt is really not the same thing.

She works part, part time, you work 24/7.

She loves to cook, you hate the kitchen unless you're decorating it.

She's basically depressed. You're on the manic side of the continuum.

She LOVES camping. You like to hike as long as the trail leads to a 5 star hotel . . .

She dresses in Gaiam yoga pants, you shop at every boutique you find while on the road.

Just a little different?

But opposites attract don't they?

OK, but make up your mind. You just were trying to tell people you were two peas in a pod, but one of you is a pea and the other is a pomegranate . . .

# CHAPTER FOUR
## "The Stalker"

*"That's the signpost up ahead—your next stop, the Twilight Zone!"*

## The Best Friend Discussion

One day after several months of everyday contact, we had a serious talk about the desire to have a best friend. We were sitting across from each other nursing soy lattes feeling very comfortable with each other. Jill looked up at me with her big soulful eyes and said she'd always wanted to have a very special friend. My ears perked up as my heart quickened a little, but I maintained a calm listening presence trying to disguise my inner elation.

She explained that while she was friendly with a number of women, they were more casual types of relationships—other mothers at school, people she spoke with briefly after a yoga class, women in the coaching program she had been a part of, old acquaintances from work. There were a number of them, but no one was that *special* person. She also lamented that she didn't understand why these other women did had their own best friends, while she struggled with finding the right one for her.

I nodded slowly, smiling encouragingly while inside my cheerleader side was waving flags and doing cartwheels yelling, "Me! Me! Here I am. Ready to go. Let's play!"

Then, she went on to talk about a "stalker" friend relationship she'd had the year before, which left her gun shy. At first, they got along great, had lots in common, enjoyed doing the same things, yada yada, but then the other woman became overly attached and wanted to be with her all the time. She was so obsessed with Jill that she was actually planning to buy a house in the same community where Jill and her husband had a retreat.

As she described the other friend, her eye brows drew together and her eyes blazed. Her whole face changed, lines from nose to mouth deepened, face flushed, jaw jutted out a bit.

Whoa!!! That woman was over the top, I silently commiserated with her even as my stomach tightened and worry began to bloom in my mind.

Her face softened as she registered what appeared like anxiety, maybe a little guilty for telling me, but then the red flush returned to her cheeks as she spat out a contemptuous analysis of this needy woman. Dana was sucking her energy, badgering her with requests to do this and that—go to the movies, go for a hike, try a new yoga studio, have dinner with both their families, go to a concert together, and a myriad more demands that made Jill want to step back, way back and reconsider their friendship.

She took a deep breath and slumped back in her chair looking spent, as if she had just finished a 50 mile bike trip. She felt drained by Dana. It was finally over and she was relieved.

Hmmmmm, I thought silently as I kept smiling and nodding to encourage her to keep talking.

Why is she telling me this? It sounds a little dangerous.

Is she warning me?

Does she see me like this other woman, Dana?

Have I been asking too much?

Have I been contacting her more than she wants?

I could be that stalker friend who wanted to be with her all the time. Up until now, it was all just a lot of fun and such a relief from my everyday working life. We painted together. We wrote together, editing each other's documents. We walked together.

And we always laughed together.

That was probably the best part. I didn't want to lose that. I couldn't lose that after having found it. It was . . . magical. How could I consider messing up a such an enchanted connection?! We were fated, weren't we? Didn't we know from that first moment? My eyes don't spark like that at total strangers. Not at people I know well, either.

And every time I ran into her after that first time, my breath hitched and I felt a little tongue tied. Really? What the hell? I'd feel a growing warmth in my chest and a smile splitting my face in half. Like the time I walked into Coffee Quest and saw her looking at an earring display. She looked up at the same time and our eyes caught and widened. "Oh Hi!" we called in chorus which led to a 10 minute conversation on how much we liked Holly Yashi designs but couldn't justify the cost, before we said, "nice to see ya" and parted ways.

Or the time we found ourselves in a meditation class with a woman who was supposedly inspired. She looked at us and told us we had deep connections from many lifetimes. That in fact we had been brothers in the lost continent of Lemuria. Lemuria? Really? I'd heard of Atlantus and Mu but Lemuria? Okayyyy. Jill and I caught eyes and giggled together. Brothers? Well, okay. Whatever.

But it wasn't until being thrown together in the weekend workshop that we actually pursued the connection further. I mean, being exposed to chocolate in small doses is manageable, but 2 straight days of constant temptation? It was just too much to not dive in.

A long time ago, my nutritionist friend, Keira, accompanied me to a set of focus groups where we were discussing some form of new protein bars. She sat in the back room along with my client from Kraft as a consultant for the creative process of designing the next generation bar.

Focus Groups are known for having huge bowls of M&M's in the backroom, in addition to other food items. But the M&M's are always the most popular. At the end of the night, Keira, who hadn't touched chocolate in years, confessed with glazed over eyes and rapid speech that she had personally downed 2 whole bowls of M&Ms to her horror and delight. It took her hours and hours to calm down enough to fall asleep after her candy coated chocolate binge. "I just couldn't resist," she moaned when we discussed it again the next day.

And now here we are, me and Jill, for better or worse and I'm not willing to put down the bowl of M&Ms? Am I binging and she's feeling consumed?

Better back down, I told myself. Put on your Psychologist hat and "treat" her if you want to keep this friendship, stay in this relationship.

So that was what I did.

I backed off quite a bit from what I wanted to do—by not being the first to reach out each day; waiting for her to contact me first. I worked on listening even more than I had been and trying to help her with . . . well, whatever she needed help on, which usually had to do with an altercation with a family member or friend or school or someone in the community. It was nice in a way. She told me all her stories and I listened sensitively, compassionately.

BUT I was "treating" her in service of our friendship. And if I had been truly treating her, if I were really her counselor, therapist, coach, it would not have been an everyday deal. We would have had appointments that were far less frequent. I would have been encouraging her to be more on her own. So rather than treating her, I was nurturing her, mommying her the best way I could, while avoiding making too many demands that would sound like her old consuming friend.

It was a trap, of course. I was pretending to just be thinking about her and being a better friend. But instead I was no longer being myself for fear of alienating her, saying the wrong thing, doing the wrong thing. She was the prize and I had to constantly win her. But I suppressed that thought so I wouldn't have to rethink the relationship. I loved the fun we had and wasn't willing to give it up. If it meant I had to change, then I would. And I rationalized it by telling myself "the only one you can change is yourself, right?"

But when you twist yourself into a pretzel or some other consumable that is palatable to another person but no longer feel like you can breathe, or eat because the cincher you've donned is so tight . . .

Sometime after that conversation and after our typical texting and giggling and ranting and commiserating, we again met at our coffee shop. She was talking about an experience with her 'best friend' . . . not me.

Her best friend!?!

Why haven't I heard about this person before?

I froze in time and attention not hearing what else she was saying except something about her best friend, who was NOT me. My head snapped back on my neck as a jolt of an electric charge surged across the table, heading down my spine, sending me spinning off into outer space, only half listening in disbelief. Ground control to Major Tom. "Uhhh . . ." was the only utterance I was capable of making in response as I continued to nod and smile like a porcelain doll bobble head with a detached body.

I was having difficulty breathing, my mouth was dry and I was instantly and simultaneously silently criticizing and judging myself for having such an intense reaction.

What was wrong with me? Jealousy? We're girls!

This is not a love—sex relationship. Why should I be feeling so . . . unimportant, uncared for, ridiculous for thinking I was more to her? I felt embarrassed to myself for misunderstanding. I was almost nauseous, ready to regurgitate all the nice things she had said to me about how she really loved having me in her life.

At the same time, I continued trying to look as though I was listening, nodding to the rhythm of her talking, smiling . . .

After a while, she came out of her self-absorbed ramble with her story and noticed that I had become a "little" pulled back. I was ready to vomit but all she saw was a disconnected stare and plastic grin.

She asked if anything was the matter. I said, "No", thinking about how at any moment I could be turning into her ex-"stalker."

She pursued and pursued.

"You look weird. What's the matter? What's going on. Sharon, are you there? Earth to Sharon . . ."

And under the tirade of questions and insistent intensity of her wide eyed distress, I blurted out my surprise and hurt about her "best friend."

The disbelief and astonishment spurted out of my mouth like a garden hose that hadn't been turned on for awhile and had explosive air pockets that forced the water out.

"Best friend?!" "What best friend?"

"But, you told me you don't have a best friend!"

"Why am I just hearing about this now?"

"What about me? If she's your best friend what am I doing here, anyway?"

Tears welled up in my eyes. I couldn't make eye contact. I felt shame. I had ruined it. I knew it. She would never be able to handle me sounding like her stalker girl.

But instead, she seemed horrified that she had upset me and immediately retorted,

"You??? You are so much more than a friend!!!! You are my soul sister! We are so deeply connected. I've never felt so understood by anyone. You really get me."

At first I felt relieved. I blinked away the tears that welled up in my eyes. Soul sister. That WAS better than a best friend wasn't it?!

Right? Maybe? What was I, a 14 year old?

Maybe. Maybe not.

Jill had been telling me about this other best friend—without the designation—for some time. She was someone that tortured her, put her down, and didn't take her feelings seriously, publicly made fun of her. What kind of friend does that? Certainly not a best friend in my world.

Jill had come to me for validation of her experience and feelings when the barbs were posted on her Facebook page. I was kind of shocked that she had someone in her life that could be that nasty and negative.

AND, I also felt superior. I'd never do that to someone I cared about.

Jill would recognize that I was really her best friend after awhile. I put it aside for the time being and reminded myself that I was better than a best friend; I was her SOUL SISTER.

Can you hear the music in the background and vibrato of the deep blues singer voice articulating the words—Sooouuul Sistuh.

[How Junior High is this sounding?]

Summer came. Jill and her family go away for the school break, spending the summer at their mountain retreat a couple of hours away. I was sad that I wouldn't be seeing her for a couple of months, but knew we could text and talk on the phone. We started to plan a visit midway.

We met a week before they were going off for break. I brought little gifts for the girls to help occupy them while on vacation. As we were all hugging goodbye, Jill casually remarked that she and her 'best friend' were going away for the weekend before she took off for the summer.

Waaaah!?!

It was something they did every year for Alzheimer's research. First time I was hearing about it. Really? Or did I just forget about it. How nice, in any case.

I mean really, what's the big deal. They were doing a 100 mile bike-a-thon. Was I going to do that? And, in the heat of late June? Very probably not, but I might have considered it, if given the option. I could have driven along side with water and energy snacks if I wasn't going to ride. But more critical was the fact that she dropped it like a giant moldy water balloon . . .

Right on my head.

I felt . . . stunned, humiliated for being caught with dripping hair and soaked shirt, and in front of the same child who had murmured, "Mommy, maybe she's the one . . ."

Uhmmm. Well, how do I react? What do I show of myself? What should I say that could possibly mediate the horrible feelings coursing through my heart and stomach and this supposedly simple "see ya soon."

We had told each other we always wanted to be open and honest, especially about our feelings, even if, PARTICULARLY if they were irrational. She must have seen my stricken expression. I'm not good at holding back my feelings on my face, unless of course, I'm in session and the coach or therapist. At that point, I was afraid to say what I felt. I kind of gulped down my emotions, wished her a good trip and asked her to send pics and text. She said she would.

I stood outside of my car and waved as she and her buckled up kids settled into their mini-van. I couldn't help thinking that I must have looked like my mother when I left her house, slow wave, edges of mouth turned down, brows up, seemingly moist eyes . . . I always felt sad and guilty like I wasn't supposed to ever leave. I hated that, not being able to leave with a happy send off. Yet, here I was doing the same to my best friend in the world?!

Jill waved back absently as she donned her sunglasses, flashed an automatic smile, took a left out of the parking lot, focused on the road ahead, and took off for points south.

That weekend, I kept looking for messages.

Well, actually, to be totally truthful, I started checking my texts almost immediately after she pulled away. She had Siri and could talk text if she wanted to. But she didn't . . .

I had become the stalker friend, overly lurking. The next day, I got a couple of texts saying she was having a great time, but tired. Who wouldn't be?

Then nothing . . . No response to my upbeat texts that were cheering her on.

Two days later, she posted a picture of herself and her best friend on Facebook in a huge triumphant embrace at the end of the bike-a-thon. Yay, them!

Well . . . REALLY, yay them! But, not yay us or yay me.

I felt abandoned, dismissed, left out, like I must be awful for her not to tell me ahead of time that she was taking this trip. Was she afraid I'd ruin it for her? She told me everything else. And I was her soul sister, right?

She came home that night and texted me a short text that she was exhausted and would be in touch the next day. I wished her sweet dreams.

The next day was the last time I connected with her for 2 months. We texted Hi, checked in with each other, and then somewhere in there I told her I was jealous.

YOW!

Too hot. Too hot, Sharon. What were you thinking?! She can't handle this! Were you thinking at all? Or, was this just little girl immaturity expressing anger and hurt, with no social filter, no impulse control?!

It was like stepping on red hot coals and feeling the fire spreading from toe to head.

She was furious, said she was going away and needed to concentrate her time on her kids and husband. AND that was that.

\* \* \*

Ohhhh no . . . . I felt awful. What had I done?! I'm trained in psychology, I coach, and I help people with their relationships all the time. What the hell! How could I have been so insensitive and self absorbed? She TOLD me she didn't like being consumed, like her stalker friend of the year before.

Oh my God, my God. I blew it!!! I burned our Maypole to the ground. Gone were the beautiful ribbons and flowers and tribute to new beginnings. I was left standing in the cold grey ashes.

In horror of what had happened, I took a giant step back to give her space and worked on myself all summer. I felt like I had made a gargantuan mistake. I was remorseful and very self flagellating.

GUILTY!!! GUILTY as charged, the jurors in my head screamed at me. Sharon Livingston, you have been found to be over bearing, needy, greedy, imposing, selfish and . . . and just too much.

What had happened to my sensitivity? She claimed she loved me because I "got her." Got her? Clearly, I demonstrated that I didn't. I was so caught up with my own needs. If I really understood her, I would have recognized her desire for space, her fear of being overwhelmed by others' needs, her wish to be in the moment and make choices based on identifying and knowing what she desired there and then, rather than being shackled and led by another's wants. She spent most of her life responding to others' concerns, needs and expectations of her. How could I add to that fire that incinerated her soul?

I talked about it in my own analysis, with my coaches, with my husband. I journaled. I talked into my iPhone recorder while walking in the woods. I lamented in imaginary conversations with her. I threw myself into my work. I wrote her emails that I didn't send. But I still felt hopeful on some inner level. We had to be able to work this out.

Right?!

Finally, it was September. She was back from her summer with the kids. I bit the bullet and called her. At first, she seemed very cool, like the doused ashes that no longer smoldered.

I owned my possessiveness and how I had imposed it on her. I was so sorry. I had no right to make assumptions about what she could or could not do with anyone else.

She said that she often would think about something that happened and wondered what I would say, how I would have understood and what suggestions I might have made. That made me teary inside as I smiled to myself feeling grateful that she still valued me.

We talked about what had happened. Or I guess I should say I asked for forgiveness for what I did. In response, she paused as I anxiously waited for some admission from her of her part in the equation.

Instead, she very seriously asked me if I was gay.

Waaaaaah?! Really?

Now, that was a stopper.

Does loving someone of the same sex mean I want to have sex with them? Really?!

But, being the seriously introspective and brutally honest with myself type, I felt obligated to ask myself the question. I thought about it seriously.

She's beautiful. I could see why guys would be attracted to her. I could see how girls would be attracted to her. So I tried to imagine what it might be like. I thought of my hubby who I do appreciate in that way. AND, well, it just wasn't what I wanted from her.

I wanted a friend, a playmate, a confidante, a collaborator, an audience for my humor—A friend who was also a woman with the special kind of nurturance that happens between female friends.

So, I said, No.

That seemed to clear the air.

We then both talked about missing each other. She said she found herself wanting to pick up the phone, and reach out to me so many times, but feared the repercussions and demands. That made me cringe a little, but I was encouraged that she was talking from her feelings and was moving towards me again.

We made peace. Not even sure how it happened, but we said nice things to each other, talked about how much we missed each other, talked about things we'd been holding in with no one to discuss them with in the same way, and I think we both felt relieved.

Over just a couple of weeks, we were back to having our texts and talks and tears and jokes, contemplating important questions, and laughing together at the follies of the world.

Over the months we painted together, shared vegan recipes, problem solved, and went back to being soul sisters.

I listened a lot and did my best to help when I could.

Even though we told each other we were bonded for life—she sent me a picture of two very old ladies walking arm in arm, smiling—I was a little worried [well maybe a lot] about asking too much, wanting too much, caring too much . . . so I remained a little cautious, sometimes tip toeing around anything to do with her relationships.

Jill would sometimes talk about others weighing her down, that she over gave and then, exhausted and drained, needed to back off, but felt guilty. At the same time, she would always point out that she wanted ME to tell her everything; to share what was happening for me, not to hesitate to call if something was bothering me, that it was different with me. While others could be draining, I nurtured and fed her, I understood in a way no one ever had. She wanted me to count on her, let her know when I was having a hard time, just like she did with me.

She actually confided in me that she understood when I felt jealous of her going away for the weekend with the other friend. When she thought about it, she realized she would have felt the same. I felt even more relieved and validated.

Still, I was cautious about the possibility of taking advantage. I thought she probably meant it when she said she wanted me to tell her my struggles and reveal my uncomfortable feelings when they came up. She did seem sincere. And at the same time I was afraid of her being overburdened. I mean, I'm trained in psychology, I'm intuitive; I can read between the lines, right?

The balance was way off, but I didn't care. I was just sooooo happy to have her back.

Was this working out, now? Could I trust that we were repairing? I so much wanted to make our friendship, our sisterhood work.

[Sigh]

Questionable!

# CHAPTER FIVE
## "Is There a Tooth Fairy?"

### The Day of the Tooth Fiasco

Did you ever have a nagging tooth that wasn't quite an ache, but just wasn't right? Kind of irritated and sometimes sensitive to cold or you feel it when you bite down.

I had a back molar that was acting up like that. After several visits to my regular dentist over a period of a number of months, he finally recommended a specialist who did an advanced laser treatment that could save the tooth. It meant Novocain and serious time in the chair.

I was literally trembling on the way to the dentist office. I know it sounds silly, but I'm highly dentist phobic, even though I see a hygienist every 3 months to clean and protect my teeth. I'm all about prevention over treatment. I take lots of vitamins to avoid having something go wrong and needing medication. I see a naturopathic doctor who is also a bio-chemist as my regular physician. It's all about wellness.

But sometimes . . .

Anyway, Jill was out of town. Her husband had left on a 2 week business trip out of the country. She seemed anxious and uncomfortable about his going and decided to take the kids out of school a few days before spring break and go on a road trip.

Truthfully? To me, It seemed extreme, but who am I to question. I mean, was it good for the kids to be taken out of school so she'd feel less lonely? What about her clients? I don't know . . . We all do some weird things when we feel abandoned and lost.

They left a day before her husband was scheduled to fly and got on the road. We checked in with each other, text, pics. I think we spoke on the phone once. Seemed like she was occupied and having a good time with them, girl bonding and sight-seeing. I thought that was great.

So, Thursday morning, as I was on the way to the dentist, having a pretty serious anxiety attack and feeling ridiculous about it, I decided to call her. I called and left a message. Twenty minutes later I called again. When there was no answer I hung up.

I was particularly nervous this time. I think I was afraid of both the effects of the Novocain which always exacerbated my anxiety response AND the possibility of losing my tooth. That COULD happen! Nothing had worked so far. AND, to make matters worse I would have to take a course of antibiotics which always made me feel lousy even when I took probiotics to counter balance them. Yech!

And I couldn't get in touch with my best friend, who promised to be there for me when I was in any kind of need. I was ALWAYS there for her like that. Right? Was it too much to ask, just this once?

But time waits for no woman.

I found myself in the endodontist's office, silently shivering in my chair in the waiting room, while the overly cheery receptionist blathered about the weather and the latest episode of Games of Thrones. [Games of Thrones? Ugh. Violent, primitive, abusive to women. What kind of visit was this going to be?]

An hour later, after I survived the procedure—which was actually surgery!—I found out I had to live on liquids for 10 days, started my Z-pack antibiotic and I unsteadily went back to work to distract myself.

My mouth was wadded with a bloody cotton ball that I had to apply pressure to. I was still numb but forewarned about pain. I had an Rx for a serious medication but I didn't want to take pain killers . . . well I just didn't. After hearing the horrible side effects in over 50 focus groups I had led on various narcotic based medicines, I wanted no part of them. I'd rather live with the discomfort and crankiness.

Over the next day I got a couple of messages from Jill—sorry about my tooth, hoped the procedure went well, that I was feeling better, had so much to share about her adventure, couldn't wait to talk. The last time I heard from her was on Friday evening. Then nothing over the weekend . . . .

I kept checking my messages, my voice mail. Nothing. I was worried.

She had confided in me that she was nervous driving in a different city, the kids were demanding, and then she went on radio silence.

On Sunday afternoon, I sent her a note, that said something like, "How are you . . . ?"

No response for hours.

So, I sent another note that said, "Hey I'm a little nervous that I haven't heard from you. Let me know how you're doing."

Nothing.

Now I was really worried.

Remember, we texted every day, multiple times per day. She's alone with the kids in a different, unfamiliar city. Is she ok? What would I do if she needed help? I was getting more anxious and concerned.

Monday came. Again nothing! On Tuesday morning, I called and left a sunrise message and then went to the gym and back to work. I had a schedule full of meetings all day long, that I had to attend to.

As I was about to start my 10 am session, my cell phone rang. I saw it was Jill and excitedly picked up the phone.

"Hiiiii How are you? How was your trip? I can't talk long right now because I have to start a Skype meeting, so I only have a couple of minutes. Is everything OK . . . ?"

She started haltingly, but deliberately. "Well, there's something that's NOT ok. I was thinking about you over the trip because I had time to think by myself and . . . well . . . Sharon, **YOU HAVEN'T CHANGED!**", she blurted out. "You're still jealous and you said you were nervous. I have a lot to do now, Jim is home, and we're going away for the weekend."

I think I felt like, sounded like Woody Allen. "I said I was nervous? But, I don't understand . . . what . . . ?"

Then my Skype call was coming in. "Jill, I'm so sorry, I have to start this meeting."

While I was on the Skype call, I sent her a defensive text saying something stupid, like I thought she misunderstood about my saying I was nervous . . .

And then total silence.

Nothing . . . .

Nada . . . .

What just happened? I was silently moaning to myself.

I felt gross, dirty. She had time by herself, thought about our friendship outside the web of my "stickiness" and decided I was bad for her? That I was trying too hard to hold on to her; I was too possessive, too intrusive, holding her back? From what? What was I stopping her from doing?

I noiselessly screamed inside from panic, frustration, incredulity, fear, self recrimination. What am I going to do? What am I going to do? What can I do? And, and why do I want to do anything? This is the second time she's pulled away? How many times do I need to be dumped to get it?!

I smelled an acrid distasteful scent. My nose searched around for its source, head swiveling side to side, up and down, lip curled, eyes squinting as if I didn't want to see the smelly offender. And then, I found it. OMG! It's me. A cold repugnant sweat is exuding from my arm pits. UGHHHH!!!

It only happened to me once before when I was going on an important job interview in my early 20's. I was wearing what I thought was a cute and chic professional dark blue suit appropriate for such purposes. Actually, it was my only suit. I really wanted the job.

It was in the city where the big girls worked. It was offering a great salary and it was for a large advertising agency with lots of opportunity to grow. AND I was recommended.

I must have been incredibly nervous, because when I entered the giant glass doors leading to the reception area and saw the beautiful woman behind the desk, I started to leak, just like now. I wasn't exactly aware of it, until I was brought into a magnificent corner office executive suite to meet two men who were there to interview me. When I reached out my arm to shake hands with one of them, that same biting stench that assaulted nostrils from 10 feet away emanated from my arm pits.

Reallllly?! What must they think? How could this woman come here without bathing. Disgusting. No Way she's stepping a foot back here ever again. At least that's what I thought they were thinking. I stammered through the short interview and left as quickly as possible.

* * *

The suit was so permeated with my off putting sour secretions that I had to throw it away. No amount of dry cleaning was able to remove it. I later learned more about it after a casual door knob comment at my next doctor's appointment. You know, that question as your walking out the door, like "Oh doc, by the way, I've been kind of constipated . . ."

In this case, it was "Oh doc, by the way, did you ever emanate a scent so vile that it would have warded off Godzilla?" He laughed and explained it was a natural protective mechanism of the body to warn off potential predators, making them want to retreat.

So here I was again, protecting myself? Even though I was alone in front of my computer with just a couple of dogs in the room, who didn't seem to take notice? And actually if they did, it would have made me more interesting to them.

They're like little kids, right? I remember having my little 7 year old niece with me a number of years ago. This is really embarrassing but . . . I was in the kitchen making something to take to my brother's house, her father. I don't cook very often. Not one of my talents. This was one of those exceptions, when I was trying to be like the rest of the family—food obsessed. I guess I had been doing too much tasting, or mixing of foods and my tummy was gurgling. At one point, one of the toxic little bubbles escaped as Jennifer was walking into the kitchen.

"Noooooo!" I was waving my arms like a gorilla gone gonzo. "Don't come in here right now!!!"

"Why?" she cocked her head and sniffed.

OMG! Really? Howwwwww embarrassssssing. And the more I asked her to leave, the more she sniffed. I must have turned scarlet, but to her it was just . . . interesting.

After tearing off my top, jumping into the shower and donning whatever was handy, I went into numb, zombie mode for the rest of the day, doing whatever was in front of me, trying to appear alive as I spoke with, coached and counseled people. Somehow I got away with it. It's amazing how much just listening and nodding can affirm someone and help them think through their own solutions.

My mind kept drifting . . . .

I thought about what happened over and over and over.

That night, over a shabby supper, my Psychologist Husband said that perhaps I sounded like a controlling Jewish Mother when I said I was "nervous". [Thank God we don't have kids!!!]

When I spoke with my mentor several days later, he agreed that I probably made her feel bad when she was trying to be grown up and off from the mother ship. He suggested that I might have said something like, "Hi. Hope you're having lots of fun with the kids. Talk soon." and leave it at that.

I felt awful. Was this my doing? Did I deserve total excommunication because I was a little worried? Or was it more like controlling and suffocating like my mother was? I couldn't step a foot out of the house without her pulling on that imperceptible pinch collar. She'd reel me in with guilt in the guise of her wondering about what I was up to. And feeling worried was a normal, protective mother quality in service of my welfare, right? I'd be pulling at my collar, hating anything tight around my neck. I felt like I couldn't breathe, hyperventilating into panic attacks.

I never wanted to be that kind of mother. UGH!! So much self-recrimination . . . . No wonder Jill pulled away. It was a natural response to being over crowded, right? Any normal person would balk at being tethered.

I actually felt a little hopeful. If it was because of my overbearing nature, I could change. I could do something that would allow her to see the real me; the real Sharon who just wanted to be her friend and was so willing to work on myself in service of our friendship. That was a great quality in a friend, right?!

I've been working on my psychology my whole life. I'm committed . . . I've always been . . . to working through my own BS, to cleaning up my act. I felt fresh and pure, like I had just stepped out of from an exhilarating and refreshing natural water fall, removing all emotional debris and tackiness.

I had evolved, right? Without those little suction cups on my fingers maybe we could shake and return to peace talking.

* * *

It's been a couple of weeks since I've written. I've been on auto pilot just going through the motions, but feeling sick inside at least part of each day, wondering what to do, as if "doing" something would/could make it better. I chose to hug myself and stay quiet, at least for a while. I wanted to honor Jill's need for space. It

SHARON LIVINGSTON, Ph. D.

wasn't my need, but I knew it was hers. In between I worked out, talked to clients, wrote, zombied out in front of the TV cuddled up to my hubby and petting the poochies.

Today, Glenn needed a "client" to demonstrate some questioning techniques for the coaching program, so he asked me to volunteer. We frequently create podcasts to teach, illustrate, motivate. Sometimes he's the coach or consultant. Sometimes I am. It's a lot of fun in addition to being informative and helpful. We work well together, a little like George and Gracie or Lucy and Desi, not quite Key and Peele, but we are often entertaining in our repartee and husband and wife flirtations.

I decided to call myself Lucy, needing something silly to counterbalance the distress. The set up is Lucy has contacted Glenn knowing that he's a relationship coach.

Lucy: Thank you for seeing me.

Glenn: Oh, hi Lucy! I was looking forward to it.

Lucy: Thanks.

Glenn: Tell me what's bringing you to me today. What can I help you with?

Lucy: I have to tell you that I feel really weird about it because, I've had couples counseling with my husband and that seems to make sense. We talked to a Relationship Coach both before we got married and during our marriage, but I'm currently having trouble with a friend. It's embarrassing to have to go and get help with a friend.

Glenn: Oh, what was it that brought it to a head that made you want to come in despite that embarrassment?

Lucy: [Heavy sigh] I thought things were getting better but I realized that they're not. Either I have to let it go or have to figure out how to make it better. Honestly, I'm not 100% sure which is the better thing to do although I'm leaning towards letting it go.

Glenn: uh huh . . .

Lucy: I haven't had a really close girl friend in a long, long, long, long time. Like really long time, maybe 10 years, 12 years, something like that. I really like having a good friend. It's really rewarding to have someone to talk with, play with, in a girl way. Someone who you can listen to and be heard, laugh with, talk about girl stuff, you know.

Glenn: Well, actually I don't, but I hear what you're saying.

He smiles encouraging me to go on.

Lucy: My husband and I are very close, but that's just different. He's really my best friend but girl talk is girl talk.

Glenn: How old is she?

Sharon: Georgette? In her 40's. Do I sound like I'm 15 or something?

Glenn: No, [laughing] I was just curious. What's the outcome you're hoping to achieve?

Lucy: One outcome would be, if things worked out, we'd talk frequently, text, and it would feel really comfortable. We'd joke and laugh a lot. We'd all get together—husbands, her kids, my niece and nephew—watch movies, play games, paint, hike. It'd just be really comfortable. We'd be there for each other.

Glenn: What was the closest you've come to having a really good buddy?

Lucy: This relationship right now.

Glenn: Our coaching relationship right now? [he tries to look serious, but a little smirk is pulling at his lips]

Lucy: Well, no, no. The woman that I'm talking about.

Glenn: I see. With Georgette?

Lucy: Yeah. I've had friends before but they were always lacking in a way where I'd end up being the caretaker, listening to their issues, and being quiet. I'd put on my shrink hat. This is soooo embarrassing to be going through, when I help so many other people with their relationships. I'm kind of cringing.

Glenn: Therapists are human too, right?

Who did you really like to spend time with when you were younger? Who was it that made you happy?

Lucy: It's not one of the things I'm really great at.

Glenn: Okay. It's almost like you're looking to fill a hole in your life.

Lucy: Wait . . . My sister.

Glenn: Your sister?

Lucy: Yeah. I did feel happy spending time with her . . .

Glenn: Tell me about her. What's her name?

Sharon: Gladys.

Glenn: Now, you have a big smile on your face.

Sharon: I've always laughed at her name.

Glenn: Did you guys laugh a lot together?

Sharon: Oh my God, yeah. We still do.

Glenn: How often do you talk to her?

Lucy: It's somewhat erratic. We'll talk everyday for a few days in a row, then sometimes not for weeks. I live here and she's down south. But we always pick up where we left off.

Glenn nods silently, inviting me/Lucy to continue.

Lucy: There is an element of me being the caregiver for her, also. But lots of times, we can laugh together. We're really honest with each other, I have to say that. We say what's really happening. I like that. If I needed something, she would do it.

Glenn: Are there one or two other things that stand out that were really stellar memories like that with her where you laugh or you just felt really bonded with her and comfortable in an integrated way, the way that you're telling me your goal is here today?

Lucy: We could be extraordinarily silly together and laugh our heads off. I'm thinking about this one time. We were in a different city on a research project. We worked together for awhile. We went into the bathroom. We each went into a stall and I let her talk to me, but I didn't answer. So people thought she was just talking . . . [Laughter] you know to herself. A crazy lady, in a stall talking to herself . . .

Glenn: That's, that's pretty funny.

Sharon: She wanted to kill me. She absolutely wanted to kill me because I just stopped talking. I let her go on and on and on and I didn't reply.

Glenn: I see.

Lucy: She didn't say anything particularly embarrassing or personal, but it was just kind of funny to hear someone sitting on the potty and talking.

She came out and said, "You, you, I can't believe you did that to me!" Then we laughed, we just laughed really, really, really hard.

She's easy to tease but I also listen to her about issues. She will tell me about anything going on in her family, with her kids, husband. I'm very, very supportive. But we can be totally, totally silly, just totally, totally ridiculous, like we were when we were little kids.

Even at this age we could make silly phone calls together or we could just be totally ridiculous until we're laughing so hard one of us would have to run to the bathroom.

Glenn: Are those the feelings that you're trying to capture and integrate into your life with a friend?

Lucy: Wowww. That's soooo interesting. You're right!

I was always called the Pied Piper of all the kids when I was growing up. I had older brothers who had children. While I was a young teenager, I had lots of nieces and nephews—14 or 15 of them. I would play games with them and entertain them. It was SUCH fun. I know how to make people laugh and play. I'm good at play. And, I practiced with my little sister.

It's actually very sweet to recognize that my sister was the model I was using.

Glenn: I have one more question for you today as we're winding down. I'm wondering, in your wildest imagination, what would have to go on here with me as your coach to help you to accomplish your goal with a friend?

Lucy: Well, I think I need a way out, an exit strategy of sorts. You need an exit strategy when you get out of a business career kind of thing, why not having an exit strategy getting out of friendship if you need to get out?

Glenn: I see. What would that look like?

Lucy: Some way of letting things go where I can still appreciate myself and not blame myself. I'm really blaming myself. It must be my fault, it must be my fault, it must be my fault.

If it doesn't work out, it doesn't work out. That has to be ok. I know that if I was helping a client, if they were telling me that something didn't work out, I'd help them dissect what happened but would mostly help them feel good about themselves.

I want to say to myself, "That's too bad. You're clearly a good person. Not that Georgette is not a good person, too, but it didn't work out. You're still good. You still have a lot of wonderful qualities. Hopefully, you'll find another playmate/friend. Maybe you will, maybe you won't. Maybe that doesn't exist in the way you're looking for it. You have a great husband, wonderful pups, a sister you can laugh with, lots of clients and friendly acquaintances. Take a breath and relax. Be nice to yourself. Chill. OK, Lucy? Ok, Lucy."

Glenn: You did a great job, Lucy. But I'd like to step out of character and debrief the session. OK?

Lucy [now Sharon]: Sure

Glenn: What was that like for you?

Lucy/Sharon: It was profound. I felt my feelings intensely. AND, I had interesting thoughts about what led up to what happened with real world Jill

I guess I'm just amazed at how important humor is to me. If you can really, really laugh with somebody, it's a representation of intimacy because you laugh at things that cause tension and stress. When you laugh really hard with someone, you demonstrate a shared understanding of each other's tensions, anxieties, frustrations, stressors. So there's a clearing of the tension with somebody who understands it and that's what happens when you can really laugh together.

It makes sense that my sister and I would have similar backgrounds with similar upsets, fears, and stressors in our lives. When we talk about something heavy at some point the humor of the situation becomes apparent and we just laugh hysterically. Not everybody deals with life like that but with you and I also, as a couple, we laugh a lot, we love to laugh.

Glenn: You could not have a friend who didn't have a sense of humor.

Lucy/Sharon: I definitely could not. Everyone in my family is kind of funny, right?

Glenn: Very funny.

Lucy/Sharon: I have a funny family and so do you. I mean your mother is hilarious.

Glenn: She is, isn't she. And, YOU are naturally very funny.

It was so interesting in working through this role play, that you were feeling that there was something wrong with you. Yet that was kind of a paradox because here you were being perfectly social and frankly, quite interesting and someone that, if I checked my own feelings, I would want to have as a friend.

Sharon: That's just because you love me and are married to me. And that's not funny, that's wonderful.

Glenn: Thank you sweetheart

Sharon: No, no! Thank you!!

\* \* \*

After my coaching session with Doc Glenn, I decided to take a chance and write Jill a short note to clear the air, take responsibility.

The first letter I wrote was overly apologetic, according to my hubby and my mentor. I basically took responsibility for everything that ever happened in the world on my shoulders. It was over the top and unnecessary. Just a simple "I'm sorry" would be better.

So after hours of rewriting and rethinking what I could/should say, that's what I did. Fingers trembling, I pushed "send" on a note that simply said,

"Dear Jill. I'm sorry. Hope all is well. Best, Sharon."

I held my breath wondering exactly how long I could live without exhalation. I was never good at doing that in beginners swimming.

I would explode out of the pool, gasping as if I'd been under water for hours.

But within seemingly no time a reply magically appeared on my screen. It was from Jill. I clicked and hungrily read the crumb of a communication.

"Thanks. We're doing great. Best, Jill."

I sat back on my stability ball, pushing back so hard that I almost fell off. [I sit on one of those instead of a chair because it's great for building core strength and I like to bounce. I have to curb it on Skype video because it can make people on the other end a little seasick sometimes. But otherwise, it's a great way to relieve stress.]

BUTTT . . . Really? That's it? My hopes for reconciliation were once again shattered.

Well, what did I expect? Clearly this is over.

But the thrashing inside my mind was reignited.

"What is wrong with her?! What kind of person can be so disconnected. Detached. This is sick, crazy, cruel. Didn't I mean anything to her?!"

"Uhmmmm. Listen to yourSELF, what is wrong with you! Do you hear yourself, so willing to blame, to name call? No wonder she pulled away!"

"Buttttt . . ."

"But what? She can only be who she is, right? Is it her fault that you read her wrong?"

I hear myself whining. "But she acted as if she really wanted to be my friend. My best friend. Her soul sister."

"You're a trained professional. You knew there were going to be problems. She gave you clues up front, right? You knew and you thought you could handle it."

"But . . ."

SHARON LIVINGSTON, Ph. D.

"But, nothing! It's not her fault. She can only be who she is. And she is NOT your friend. Not now. Maybe never. OK?"

"Since when have you become the Ugly Truth Teller?" I quip in retaliation at myself.

Then I tune in to how harsh I'm being with myself and tears well up as I allow myself to roll off the stability ball onto the floor and crumple into a fetal position, folding my knees into my chest and letting the salty hot grief and frustration drip out of my eyes.

# CHAPTER SIX
## "Downward Dog"

Time heals all wounds. Isn't that what they say? But how much time?

It's been a hard and tumultuous couple of weeks. At many moments: Miserable, depressed, angry, anxious, aimless, frustrated, despairing, wanting, conniving, sad, quiet, slightly hopeful, wanting to scream, "You are not really my mother who abandoned me over and over and made me feel it was my fault!!!" And then calmly, "it just feels that way . . . .

It's been hard to focus. I work as I always work. But, as soon as there is a break, I'm distracted wondering . . . .

. . . What if . . . ?

What if I hadn't left those last 2 texts? What if I had been more patient? What if I drove over, knocked on the door, looked in her eyes and said, "Hey it's me! Remember? We were soul sisters, right? Forever, till old ladies? Remember? You said that. You said you wanted that. I'm the same person. I'm still caring, understanding, available for you [not for everyone you know, but for you], funny and, and, and kind of pathetic." [Head down, ears down, tail between my legs, whining]

What changed? What Changed?

You did?!? You've outgrown me? Had an epiphany about relationships and friends and what you want? Really?!

You're doing the same thing you always do, when it gets too hot, you jump into the Atlantic and swim to France.

I thought it would be different with us. That you would like the closeness, even love it. That I would be soooooo unbelievably irresistible as a friend, that you would put away your fears and dive in.

It wouldn't be THAT deep! I know about fear of water. We could go into the shallows to restart and perhaps sometimes take a risk, hold hands and step through the depths on occasion, just for fun! Like an amusement park ride, where you safely face your fears of height and speed.

I do have a sense of humor. Glenn said so, right? I'm not morose. I'm a little needy. Yeah, that's true. But Glenn and I get through it. We've been married for 26 years and we know how to navigate the waters, even when they include some pretty hot tears. Isn't that what it means to be a true friend?

AND, and, you're gone, but you're not. How can I let you go knowing you're living and breathing and just down the road, with those sparkly alive eyes and with so many interests that I love to hear about, even the new tofu love casserole covered in artichoke hearts? Isn't there something I can do? Something . . . ??!!!

But no! You're alive to the world but dead to me. I have to mourn and let go. Hurts sooooo much . . . even now . . . . weeping inside with leaking, sad eyes . . . .

\* \* \*

I just can't help it. I keep analyzing and analyzing and analyzing. Going over all the details, all the signs of trouble; disconnect.

Critical Differences?

In personality theory, I'm an "E," a natural extravert getting energized by people contact. I thrive on interactions with people. She's an "I," an introvert, she likes people but can only handle so much. She reenergizes by being alone.

She has young kids, I have old dogs.

She's a career Mom, I'm a workaholic, juggling several hats and roles.

She likes to swim and bike; I like to write and hike.

She teaches yoga; I can't touch my toes.

She loves sugar and doesn't show it; I love sugar and bloat.

She . . .

She . . .

SHE CLEARLY SAID SHE DOESN'T LIKE BEING CROWDED.

Get it?

My body tenses, I again stop breathing as my inner child screams in frustration and despair.

### Out Of Balance Relationships
### Are Doomed To Fail

In talking to one of the many friends I had to unload my distress on or explode, I heard him say that the relationship was out of balance.

He's an old friend who knows my history, a college buddy. He reminded me that my part was the repetition of the anxious attachment I had with my mother.

Ooooo . . . . Hurts but was true. How is it possible that I could forget everything I know and use to help others!! How is this even possible? How can I be so astute, compassionate and a great guide for people I help, but blind to my own patterns.

Breathe, Sharon. Yes, you help others, but you're also human. Doctors stopped being gods in the 90's when Managed Care defrocked them, remember?

Yes, I wanted contact with her more than she wanted with me. I anxiously awaited any sign that she was aware of me, maybe thinking of me, wondering if I was as important to her and then shutting that thought down because I felt embarrassed to myself that I was craving any sign of recognition from her that I existed.

I was willing to do whatever it took to maintain the friendship. She had a different agenda. I made her more important and devalued myself in the process.

She became more and more creeped out by my wimpy, self effacement. Honestly, I would have felt the same way. No one wants to be around a groveling Gollum of Hobbit fame; nor the hopping-on-one-foot princess in "Coming to America," right? "Whatever for my Precious. Yes, master. Whatever you say master. Whatever you like."

As disgusted with myself as I feel when thinking of how I was willing to do anything to be her friend, it makes sense in light of my history and early development.

Babies form attachments to their caregivers as part of their need to survive. They can't exist on their own. Depending on how well attuned their caregivers are or are not, the baby/child develops behaviors and feelings about self which are carried into adulthood.

When parents are in touch with the baby's needs and validating to them in a loving way, the baby is likely to grow up with a sense of security and confidence in self. Unfortunately for many of us, that is often not the case. Or we start out trusting and some crazy life event intervenes and makes us risk averse, suspicious and either retreated and protected with a gate and lock around our hearts, or clingy and fearful.

I can see how I developed the clingy form. There I was a cute little, spirited 5 year old, trying to assert my independence by asking my mother to wait a minute when she asked me to bring her a thimble. When I dutifully returned a few minutes later than she expected, she punished me by not recognizing me. She sat sewing, refusing to take the thimble, refusing to acknowledge that I was even there talking to her, visible in the room. I repeatedly tried to give her the thimble but she was stone faced and bodied, moving mechanically except when she winced as the needle painfully probed her unprotected finger tip.

It was terrifying to me. Had I ceased to exist? It was so frightened that I started crying, begged her to talk to me, elephant tears streaming down my face. She finally put her sewing down, after I was hysterical on the floor, arms and legs flailing, sobbing, snot dripping out of my nose. She pulled herself up to her prideful full height [all of 4'9", I'm not kidding you] and stood over me like the wicked step mother in Snow White. She looked down at me with contempt, "now have you learned your lesson?" She dripped contempt.

Now that I think about it, Jill seemed to be the Lock Up Heart type while I became the begging, clingy Gollum. Pretty gross! Gollum had a love hate thing for his addictive Precious ring which reflected the love and hate he had for himself.

Heavy, man . . .

[Heavy sigh]

## Spirals of Connections

I have this image of people cycles that you might conceptualize as energy spirals like little twisters that move through the world. As they are swirling sometimes they encounter other spirals and for a time connect and swirl together. Some spirals stay in the same field for a long time, maybe forever. Others touch, swirl together for a while and then detach and go on their ways. Not a judgment, just an observable phenomenon.

## Kubler-Ross's 5 stages of grief

You've probably heard this before, so I'll be brief. Dr. Elizabeth Kubler-Ross studied dying people and those who loved them. Both the person dying and the people who loved them dearly went through a series of predictable emotional reactions:

- Denial,
- Anger,
- Bargaining,
- Depression,
- Acceptance . . . .

These same stages are evident in EVERY loss.

Denial—No! This is not happening!

Anger—at the other person—how can you be doing this? What's the matter with you? Stop it, right now! Let's go back to before when everything was fine.

Bargaining—I'm sorry. I'm willing to . . . If only I had . . . [fill in the blanks as many times as you can]

Depression—the anger and pain about the loss gets turned inward and we retreat into sadness, remorse, self-loathing, and withdrawal.

Acceptance—Recognizing that this relationship is permanently gone and we have to go on, have a good life, even though we miss the other.

Around the time that I was thinking about the 5 stages, I had a series of talks with a young single friend whose boyfriend had broken up with her. She was beyond upset. He had said very cruel things to her, blaming her for his need to leave. He told her she was stuck in her patterns and would never change.

I want you to know a few things about her. She's brilliant—an innovative thinker, organized, beautiful, caring, open . . .

As she was telling me about this rejection, I couldn't help but identify with many of the feelings she was having both emotional and physical.

She was so upset that she spent weeks feeling nauseous.

Really? Me too?! I thought it was just from the antibiotics. Hmmmm.

She felt lethargic, unmotivated to do anything but go home after work and feel lousy over the abandonment.

Me too. And, I have a loving husband! What was I doing? How must this be making him feel? Felt sooooo bad that my upset had to be affecting him too.

She started doubting herself. Is he right? Am I stuck and unmovable? What did I do? Does that mean I can do something else and we'll be ok?

Yep. Yep. I get that. Hmmmm. Should I call her? Should I send her something? Should I show up where she does and casually bump into her? NOOOOO! Stay put! Sit still. Just feel without acting! Can you do that? OMG, this is the hardest thing, to DO nothing . . .

I still love him. If he calls me, I'll want to be with him.

Ugghhh. He was so rejecting. Why would she still want to be with him? She had told me so much about him that made me want to put a permanent security guard around her so he couldn't get close to her.

And, at the same time, I knew that if Jill reached out to me, I would be there in a flash. Ughhhh. Why would we do that to ourselves when it was a clear set up for another rejection?! This wasn't the first time he'd hurt her. Wasn't the first time Jill had shut-down! Fool me once shame on you. Fool me twice, shame on me. How many times do we have to be left to realize we'll be tortured again?

So, yeah, I can see the 5 stages of Grief playing out:

Denial: This isn't really happening. She'll get in touch with me in a few days. Just be patient and give her space. Fingers strum, strum, strum, strum . . .

Anger: What is wrong with her! After all I've done for her!!! She's selfish, narcissistic, and afraid of friendship, immature . . . Ugh. Am I describing myself? Am I seeing my worst qualities projected onto her? And, if so what do I do with that? I'm nauseous again . . .

Bargaining: Listen, what is it you want? I can do it. It's ok if I never ask for anything, just to be with you sometimes, and listen to you, help you figure "it" out, whatever that is, I'm great at that. Remember that old ad—"Let me be your Brill-o pad". "If you love me you'll use me."

Depression: Ugh, do I have no self-worth? Am I really willing to do anything? To buy friendship?! What does that make me?! Do I have no values?! Do I have no self-worth?! And, what is wrong with me that I would choose such an unfruitful friendship?! I'm just not good enough—too dependent, needy, insecure, stupid for having made such a bad choice. Mom was right. Now look what you've done! And, I'm taking away from my husband, not being present as I can. This is mean to him. Ughhh. What is wrong with me?!!!!

After my young friend had time to tell me about her ex, I shared with her that I had just gone through something similar with a female friend. After I shared some of the details, she said, "Ohhhhhh, losing a girlfriend like that is even worse . . . ! It's such a total betrayal. It's worse than a loss of passion and romance. You can kind of understand when a guy and gal don't work out, but two friends?! That's a heart connection that's not supposed to be broken. It doesn't need sex to keep it alive; it's about recognition of another human being—kindred soul and acceptance of your heart print. You feel like you're connected for life. You must feel awful!!!"

I did. I do.

I shared with her about the 5 stages of loss.

The way it's usually talked about makes it seem linear. You start with Denial and walk through the stages till you get to acceptance and moving on with your life.

But it's NOT linear. It's more like that spiral. You can move through the stages again and again. Just when you think you're through, something reminds you and you're caught up again, swirling in their space, sometimes angry again. Or you forget about the separation as the recalled energy pattern appears to sweep you round and round and think to yourself, oh, I have to tell Jill about . . . but you can't. You're twirling solo, arms raised and poised atop non-existent shoulders. She's in a different force field; one where you don't exist. And then the depression and grief hits again.

It takes longer than you think to move along this emotional conveyor belt. Mourning someone who's died must take at least a year; a year to go through all the seasons without that person in your life, a year to make new associations and memories that no longer include the past relationship. But when the person is alive and real and living in your local vicinity . . . there's always hope, a wish that something will change, that she'll get religion and realize the errs of her ways, that she'll see me for the—interesting, intelligent, caring, witty, intuitive, entertaining, compassionate, [fill in the blank] friend that I am and want to start again . . .

UGH. There have been other examples where I got sucked into the dance and stayed and suffered the ups and downs of the deadly tango for years. As painful as it was, is . . . This time, no strike three.

# CHAPTER SEVEN
"The Beat Goes On"


I feel the resolve. It's time to get up from the table. The band went home hours ago. The bus boys are folding up the chairs. The bartender is trying to catch my eye as he nods toward the door. It's almost dawn

It's a new day. I've had my coffee and I'm back behind my Mac, on my stability ball, symbolically dusting the dry crumbs of nutrition-free toast off my skirt. I take a deep breath and look up with determination to move on, a little bit of an upbeat feeling travels up my torso as I cheerlead myself.

So what now? What else do I have to say? Feel? Do?

Time heals all, right?! It's been weeks since this upheaval in my life; I'm actually beginning to lose count of the days.

Let's do it, team! I stand and clap my hands together, flashing a smile at myself in the mirror above my desk. I'm going to do my work out, my 100 flights of stairs, shower and get dressed in something sweet.

I kick off my shoes, head over to the foyer and start my ascent—up two flights—down two flights, up two flights, down . . .

As the air fills my lungs to help propel me up, I remind myself that I encourage myself. I could rehash and rehash and probably will somewhere, but **not here anymore**.

As much as I'm complaining, refusing to want to accept that Jill and I are no more a friendship, I can go on, I will go on, Look, I AM going on—doing what I do every day, climbing my stairs, feeling strong and capable. How many people do 100 flights of stairs 6-7 days a week?! Look at you! I smile to myself as if I'm encouraging a little girl who's learning about the value of exercising her strengths and growing.

I muse to myself, you know . . . Glenn and I are actually a little closer. He's been compassionate and sweet. He's listened, commiserated and held me. He has a best bud and would be crushed if that relationship suddenly ended.

I've returned to putting emphasis on my work, which I love. My pups . . . . Maybe I'll find my diamond now that the snow has finally thawed.

AND, I'm using this experience as an opportunity to work through whatever it is that Jill represents to me on as many levels as I'm capable.

I'm an optimist at heart and believe that something good will come of this.

Dear Jill,

What I wish for you and for myself is clear sight and an open heart and taking our time to forge enduring friendships.

To Friends!! Whoever, whenever they may be.

# CHAPTER EIGHT
## "The Abyss"


I haven't written in a couple of weeks. Don't know why. Wanted to avoid the topic even though it goes round and round in my mind, circling down to my heart and my gut, bowing my spine, weakening my muscles so I just want to go back to sleep, but can't. Thank goodness I have a life in the real world. I have to work, have to focus on the rest of my life, my husband, my pups, my students, my clients. They need me present and whole, as whole as I can be.

Can I be real and be whole? Can I be here with myself and then step out of my pain and be fully present for them? Can I be vulnerable, raw, and yet fully related to them?

It's tough. It's really tough. Even though a sense of hope peeps out at me from the sunlight behind the curtains, I fight the feeling of wanting to close my eyes and dip down into the heaviness of dejection and gloom.

Why would I choose to go there, to roll over and bury my head in my pillow? And, is it a choice? Do I really have control? Am I wallowing in self-pity? I hate that in myself and in others. Nothing good comes out of self-pity, does it? Self-pity means that I'm seeing myself as a victim, without blame or responsibility of the consequences. Self-pity is denial that I could have created this mess.

BUT . . . If I recognize that it's my own doing, if I admit I made a terrible mistake, will I get punished? Will I get hit, beaten? Like a ton of bricks crashing down on me? Will I be filled with humiliation . . . again? Made to feel worthless? Have to be by myself? Alone?! Isolated?! Frightened the boogie man will get me, because he preys on little girls who have to go upstairs by themselves in the dark.

My brothers whispered that to me every night when I was commanded to go to bed, "The boogie man is gonna to getcha!" I pictured a giant ugly monster made out of green dripping snot, reaching for me, laughing a deep dark derisive g-u-t-t-e-r-a-n-c-e.

Wait . . . no one else is condemning me, are they? Jill may not want to be in a relationship with me, but does that mean she's condemning me? That I've become ugly and gross and disgusting to her?

Am I condemning her?

I'm again stuck. In a quicksand of sticky tears that can't pass through my tear ducts, that collect behind my eyes and fill my head seeping down, down, stifling my voice, making it hard to breathe, like a slow whirlpool of thick sludge, drawing me to the depths, pulling on my ankles, I don't pull away, just feel trapped and gooey in this chilly determined quagmire of mud and vines and purpose . . .

Huh? I wake for a second hearing my thoughts. Purpose! What purpose?

The dead pool snarls.

"To bring you to your knees! To make you beg. To make you realize you're not worthy of living. You should be grateful. I saved your life even though I wished you had never been born. You weren't supposed to be born. You're a drag on me, on the family. We didn't need another child, want another child. So I will suck the life out of you, bring you to my grave, bring you back to where you belong, to who you really are, to nothing, to cloying sticky muck that sucks the life out of everyone else.'

A scream is stuck in my chest, never even making it to my throat, but stealing my breath as my heart pounds in terror. This voice! So disturbing, sending panic up my spine.

Making three boys was enough mud for my parents to be playing in, too much, too much for them to handle when they were children themselves.

They made a mistake. They didn't mean to get pregnant, THIS time. God knows I've heard that 100's of times. AND, AND, and then you had the nerve to be a girl!? And . . . adorable with mischievous sparkly eyes, smart, creative, and TALL?! You were the biggest baby of all the babies. What the hell were you thinking?! Why did you choose to be born to this family? What karma are you working on? Ugly Duckling! Don't embarrass me!

Oh my God, wait a second. What am I telling myself?! Why am I indulging in this exercise of victim? I'm soooo dramatic!!!

Is this cathartic . . . ?

I think it helps when I write, when I touch the depth of my feelings in language and say what comes to mind. I share this with my writing coach who listens compassionately, intently, empathetically and despite the pain of what I say out loud to myself, he shares his excitement about my ability to express.

But . . . am I ever going to be free? Free of the echoing loneliness that I've avoided, shut out, but lived with forever? Lonely in a crowd!? Lonely in my huge family!? Lonely in my own company!?

We'd have 60 people at Passover dinner when I was 5-8. So many that "I" was sent to the neighbor's house so "I" wouldn't get in the way.

Well, what do you expect!

SHARON LIVINGSTON, Ph. D.

Get it through you're thick head! You weren't welcome or wanted. Nobody wanted you there. You were demanding, dead weight, a nuisance, a drain. You always wanted something that took them away from their own needs. Remember? There were sooooo many instances of them not wanting you around. Should I remind you?!?

STOP! You're hurting me!!! This hurts. Then I collapse.

Whirlpool pools at my legs.

"Don't bother." Its deep sultry voice intones. "Stop listening.

Let me take you down.

It's cool down here.

You know how much you hate being hot.

It's cool.

You'll relax.

You'll stop being afraid.

You'll stop feeling, feeling pain, sadness, scare. You'll sleep. You'll sleep a dreamless sleep without dread, without dream."

I drift, feelings numbed for the moment.

I realized a few days ago that there was never, NEVER, a time when my mother CHOSE to spend time with me because she wanted to be with me.

NEVER!

She put up with me, had me attended to in some way—by herself or another, but NEVER wanted, desired, opted to spend time with me just because . . . Because I was cute, fun, smart, interesting . . . worthy of her love . . . of anyone's love.

Never a time when my Dad *chose* to be with me . . . and rarely spent any time with me . . . except to dole out punishment because Mom told him I had misbehaved, done something objectionable, been bad.

My grandmother would threaten, "Wait till your father comes home."

She was stuck with me because they couldn't find a nanny, because I was insufferable? [Was that my fault too?] Dad strapped me on my tender, bare butt two times that I remember. Maybe more . . . ? Is that why I wince when anyone raises their voice at me? When anyone expresses annoyance or displeasure? Because I fear I'm in big trouble, the leather strap is about to come out and strike my skin, with the burn of fire and humiliation of being undeserving of . . . ?

But the worst, worse than being beaten, is becoming a non-person. Mom never raised her voice. The angrier she became, the quieter and calmer she appeared until she was so angry that she refused to acknowledge my existence. I was invisible. No matter how I begged or cried she pretended I wasn't there.

The bog beneath me, tugs and brays in deliberate, gritty doggedness.

'Stop fighting. Stop screaming. It's futile. Then, more softly . . . let me take you down.'

# CHAPTER NINE
## "Wicked Witch of West Jersey"


Yesterday was my mother's birthday. She passed 6 years ago, but I started worrying about her dying when I was 12.

Both of her parents died within a year of each other. Her mother died at 73 of a heart attack, sitting in the kitchen on a straight backed chair, hands gently clasped in her lap and then, small gasp, toppling over and gone.

Mommy's 80 year old father died a year later after having spent much of that time living with us.

Two weeks before he passed, I had a nightmare that a door fell on him, killing him. I felt scared and guilty. Somehow it was my fault? Did I kill him with my dream? Was it prophetic or just coincidental? I didn't tell anyone because I was afraid of being seen as wicked, wishing him ill. And then he died of a blood clot. Both of my grandparents died suddenly, no one expecting it to happen. I was secretly terrified that I had caused Zadie's death with my dream.

My mother was understandably shocked and very disturbed to lose both parents in such a short span. She didn't talk about her feelings, instead somatized. She kept thinking she was having a heart attack—sharp pains in her chest. She actually spent time in the hospital with a diagnosis of some kind of heart condition.

When she came home, she retreated into what was later described as a cardiac neurosis and severe depression, although we didn't understand it at that time. Later we learned that after all the nitro-glycerin, Coumadin and beta blockers, what she'd had was a digestive disorder triggered by panic and anxiety. Why didn't they know that?! She'd had colitis for years, severe panic attacks in her 20's . . .

But, that's not my reason for bringing up Mom.

When she got the diagnosis, she started acting differently. After being a little dynamo, workhorse—sometimes working 36 hours in a row, she retreated to bed. I'd go visit her and want to cuddle up next to her. She'd tell me to go away because she didn't want me to fall asleep and wake up to find her dead.

I was horrified. It didn't occur to me until just now, writing about it, that that was how she experienced her parents' deaths. She was shocked and horrified that suddenly they were gone. She had unresolved hurts and desires with her own mother. She wanted more of being her Daddy's girl, which somewhat made up for her mother's harshness.

My mother learned to use her "heart attacks" to control my behavior. Whenever I did something she didn't like, she would have to go to bed because of the pain in her chest.

The worst was when she discovered I was no longer a virgin. I was 20. I came home from school to find Mom in her bed—her eyes were red and shiny, her breathing was labored, her lips made a steep arc with end points almost down to the bottom of her chin. She was clearly suffering. Worried, I implored, "Mom what's the matter?"

She paused, slowly turned her head to face me [like Chucky in that horror flick] and in her typical melodramatic voice with her Hungarian accent, whispered, "I know . . ." Heavy lids over pupils that stared staring piercingly into my own.

My eyes widened. I could feel the air cool and drying their surface. Frantic and guilty, I sputtered, "You know what?!"

She said nothing, turned away. And like I did when I was five and she refused to talk to me because I didn't retrieve the thimble she requested, I started begging her to tell me.

"What . . . ?! You know what?!" My heart was pounding. I felt terrified. How could she know?! After what seemed like hours but was probably only a minute, she opened her eyes, stared at the ceiling and hoarsely rasped,

"I want you to get married . . . tomorrow!"

I was in shock. I was not ready to get married, not sure what to do. AND, How could I bring up marriage to my boyfriend?!

She was kidding, right?

"Tomorrow . . . ?" I squawked, voice like a stuck chicken.

She nodded slowly but deliberately. No words.

OMG! OMG! I CAN'T get married. I don't even know if I want to marry this guy. He's always looking at other women. Always letting me know he may want to take a break.

But she could die at any minute!

What's more important, saving my mother's life or figuring out what I need for the rest of my life? She sat propped up in the bed, staring into space, every now and then grunting as she clutched her chest.

"It's just a gas pain," I screamed silently feeling my face contort. She always did this to me. Just when I was beginning to have my own life she'd reach out with her razor sharp hooks and tear at my heart, making me the cause of all her torment.

It was a Catch 22. No good answer. Reeling inside, heart hammering, feeling like the sky was falling, crushing me, I ran to her medicine cabinet, grabbed a little bottle that was used for Mom emergencies and took MY first tranquilizer.

As I was writing this, I felt a pain in my chest. Nurture or nature!? Did I inherit panic and anxiety disorder or did I learn it . . . ?

Deep breath . . . . Another . . . .

# CHAPTER TEN
## "Just Ducky"

Someone sent me the cutest video of a duck with her brood of ducklings. Momma Duck was at the top of three concrete steps that were integrated into a walking path in a public park. Her tiny offspring were heroically following her but stymied by the height of the steps. One baby made it up to the second step fairly quickly and then struggled to hop up one more to join her, but succeeded. It looked like she bowed her head to give him a little appreciative peck on his head. The two stood there, sometimes pacing along the top level, waiting for the others to arrive.

The others persisted for many failed trials, sometime falling on their tiny backs but popping back up. Mom stayed patiently above, watching sometimes, or just standing and waiting. Eventually, all of them somehow got themselves to the top of the steps to rejoin their family. Together all walked into a neighboring flower bed. It was soooo adorable and inspiring. My first thought was to send it to Jill . . .

Then I stopped in my tracks.

"No, you can't."

"But she would love it! And she'd show it to the kids and they would love it," I whined to myself.

"No."

"Why?"

"It's not appropriate. You're not friends."

"But I want to be friends," tears beginning to well up in my eyes.

Grown up Sharon drops down to meet little Sharon at eye level.

"Come here, cutie. I'm soooo sorry. I know you want to play with Jill. And the duckies are soooo adorable and fearless and Look, they did it! They were on a mission and they just kept trying till they succeeded. That's so impressive for such tiny little beings, isn't it?"

"It is . . . But I want to show Jill."

"I know. It must be awful not to be able to share it with her."

"You are so strong to share it with me and we can enjoy it together."

"Would you like to share it with someone else?"

"Yes." I say hesitantly.

"Who?" Grown up Sharon asks with a smile in her voice.

"Lisa."

"Oh what a great choice. I'll bet Lisa would love it. She loves animals and adorable babies. And she's a very persistent person herself. What a good choice. Let's go send it to her."

"Ooo Kay." Small smile . . . . "I know she'll love it, too."

# CHAPTER ELEVEN
"Can't Buy Me Love"


Got up this morning with lots on my plate! Flight to Chicago this morning was cancelled last night. In fact 350 flights were cancelled. Had to get creative to figure out how to manage our project; clients coming to observe; 15 people showing up to be interviewed. And, no way to get to Chicago today or in time for tomorrow! My Field VP and I scramble to set up a remote interview option late last night. I think it's going to be fine. Have to cancel hotel and car service. Anxiety provoking . . . . Did we miss anything? Hurry up, go to sleep.

Silver lining—I get to sleep in my own bed another night. Get to snuggle with Glenn and play with pups a little more. Get to juice vegetables which I won't be able to do on the road.

Sit down. Take a deep breath. Give myself the luxury of writing . . .

As I was thinking about sitting down to write, giving myself this time to ruminate, I realize that I was NOT obsessing about Jill this morning.

Wowwww! That's a change. I'm smiling to myself as I walk over to the refrigerator and take out a box of Cashew milk to add to my Zen tea.

Hmmmm. Feeling a little excited and relieved at the same time . . .

But wait.

I said I was NOT . . . I stop in the middle of pouring the milk into my oversized pink mug.

But here I am thinking about her again.

Yeah . . . but . . . with less pain . . . . I think I feel less pain and upset. Other things on my mind, in my life to attend to . . . my work—getting all of these interviews done well, even though they will be remote and my clients will be there while I'm a talking head, preparing the next module for our Coaching Academy, doing more here so I can finally be free to return to my biz book.

I take my mug out of the microwave, add some Stevia and bring it back to my desk. I sit down and take a deep breath, as I position myself to open my document.

Ugh. It just occurred to me. Do I think that by writing this, Jill will be so moved she'll come visit me, just like my Dad did?!

Arrrggggh.

I sit on my ball, legs straight out, arms suspended over the keyboard, but not touching. Just in a daze, realizing what I've been doing . . .

What kind of magical thinking is this, I challenge myself.

Sharon, do you think you have the power to will her by thought to seek you out? Because you're not going to mail this emotional treatise to her like you did when you sent the letter to your Dad, Right?

No. I mean I want to but I won't. heavy sigh, head down, lips curled and beginning to tremble.

AND, you're not her blood and flesh. I try to reason with myself.

You didn't live in the same house with her for 21 years. She doesn't have the same investment in you, even though you appear to have it in her.

I decide to change the subject. This is too much now and I have so much to do.

Look on the bright side. I HAVE been very involved with my students. They are complex, smart, introspective and caring people who want to give, to help others grow. Their stories of how they came to coaching are varied and fascinating, sometimes shocking, sometimes very painful, always stimulating, always fascinating, always soooo touching.

What they have in common is a passion about their particular knowledge and experience in the world. They really want to contribute what they have learned; want to help people achieve their goals and if at all possible bypass the sometimes precipitous pitfalls they themselves encountered.

While they figured out how to get back on their feet, back on the road, they wished they could have avoided the scare, the pain, the upset, and the setbacks—which at times were measured in years.

They wished there had been someone to gently guide THEM so they could have avoided the distress and move along more smoothly. . . . Like having a helpful hint page on a video game. You don't have to stay stuck, or get eaten by a monster. You CAN get help and get out of that situation so you can move ahead. You're not alone. Others have traveled this path, or a similar path. There are tricks. There are tools. There's comfort available when you get in trouble. And it's ok to run to shelter for just a little trouble. You don't have to wait till it's an avalanche.

They are so inspiring! What a gift to be working with such phenomenal human beings. It fills me with awe and I feel so lucky to be doing this work.

* * *

I break for a moment to drink some fresh juiced veggies when a wave of feelings, clenching that grabs me in the gut and rushes through my system. I double over catching my breath, pain grips my stomach, burning, nausea.

Oh God. Here I am again, thinking to myself did I mean nothing to her? NO! NO! It's not that. It can't be that. We had too much fun and talking and discussing deep issues for you to mean nothing to her. You probably meant too much. So she had to block you out.

Yeah but she blocked out that other woman she thought of as a stalker.

Decided she was crazy.

Do I sound crazy?

Am I crazy?

Obsessed? The way she talked about that other woman made her sound like someone that should be dismissed, cast out like a toxin. It made sense to me she wanted out, to avoid her, never talk to her, pull out of a parking lot if she saw her car there.

Has she seen MY car and driven the other way?

Why do I keep torturing myself?

I refocus on the positives, distracting myself.

I was just saying how meaningful my life has been working with so many inspirational people who are dedicated to creating significant practices for themselves. These are people who have faced and continue to face their demons and challenges and have survived with important stories to tell, with encouraging lessons to share, who want to make the world a better place. They have thought through their experiences and outlined a series of paths one might take to bypass the slippery slopes, mires, rocky impasses that can lead to disasters or major setbacks and delays. They are fascinating. They fill me with hope for the future. I feel sooo proud of how they learn. They're like grown up kids to me that I get to guide, watch them take in information and sculpt it via their understanding to match their personalities and communication styles. I feel satisfied like a proud mother hen.

But they are not my friends. They like me, maybe a few would say they love me, but they are my chicks. It's not the same as having a friend who I DIDN'T buy.

At first, Jill and I were equals. We just enjoyed being with each other. Neither of us was higher or lower because of a determined hierarchical relationship. We didn't work together. We had different strengths as well as wishes for growth. I didn't go to her yoga classes. She didn't work part time for me, even though we both could have benefitted in each case. We wanted to be equals. We wanted to avoid polluting our friendship with possible superimposed roles that could change things.

I find myself wringing my hands.

But there are many ways to change the balance of power, right?

# CHAPTER TWELVE
### "Telephone Puppets"

Hi Jill

OMGosh! What a day or is it two days by now . . . .

Nope, I can't do it. Thought it might be a good idea, but I feel ooky, another sinking feeling in my stomach.

* * *

A few years ago, a few years after my mother died, I was driving from Lincoln NH where our condo was located, down to Hannaford's the big supermarket in Plymouth. It's a 20-25 minute drive. It was a Sunday morning and we needed to replenish the pantry.

Glenn was working so I took Stewie and we went for a drive. I missed my mother—her soft, cool pink cheek;

her scent of old Faberge Woodhue; I wished I could call her. Reeeeeally wished I could talk to her.

So, I picked up my cell and dialed her number. I pretended that she answered and had a conversation with her, a long conversation, where I voiced both sides of the dialogue. It was pretty easy. I had been talking with her for my whole life so I knew the kinds of things she'd say. So I just filled in for her. It was actually pretty easy barring the Hungarian accent.

"Hi Mom . . ."

"Surala, how are you? I vas vondering ven I vould hear from you."

"How are you Mom? What's it like up there. How's Dad? How's everyone else?"

When she passed, I went for a cranial sacral treatment with a guy who also did Reiki energy work. He was the person who helped me reframe my experience of anxiety, so I felt safe with myself with him, safe allowing my reveries to be expressed and witnessed. I told him Mom had passed . . . . That I was in some kind of shock about it, hard to describe . . . .

\* \* \*

Glenn and I drove down to Philly where the funeral was being held. She would be buried next to my father, next to his mother and father. I've never been one to visit cemeteries, unless I had to, at such an occasion as this.

We stayed at my favorite hotel in center city where I knew all the service staff. They took care of Stewie for me when I stayed there on a work trip. Felt a little like home. That morning, Sunday morning, we got into the car, I drove, it was my car and not quite tall enough for Glenn's height, but he could put the seat back in the passenger seat.

I had the directions to the funeral parlor. Started off, slowly, carefully, recognizing I needed to be focused since this was a disturbing day. Made a left on 16th street going North towards the Ben Franklin bridge . . . and went straight through a red light.

"SHARON!!!" Glenn's voice intruded. "You went through a light!!! Are you ok to drive?"

"I'm ok, I'm ok", I felt shocked. How had that happened? I forced myself into hyper-vigilance. I wanted to drive. I needed to be in control.

I had thrown together a PowerPoint celebrating Mom. Opened the deck at the receptions area and played it on a continuous loop—the best of Mom, pics with her and Dad and my brothers and sister and cousins and aunts and uncles. Smiling, comical, sweet, the way I wanted to remember her, the way I wanted to think of her, turn her into my ideal Mom.

Even as I looked at the smiling pictures, I couldn't help remembering an old song from *Hair*.

How can people be so heartless?

How can people be so cruel?
Easy to be hard, easy to be cold
How can people have no feelings?
You know I'm hung up on you
Easy to be proud, easy to say no

And especially people who care about strangers
who care about evil and social injustice
Do you only care about the bleeding crowd?
How about a needing friend? I need a friend

Tears welled up behind my eyes, but I pushed them back, sniffed them back, shaking my head and sitting tall. I had to be strong for my little sister. So I came out of my reverie and joined her to go into the chapel where the coffin was on display. The casket was closed. The director asked us if we wanted to see her. We looked at each other. I impulsively answered for the two of us, ever taking care of her, "Yes. Thank you, yes we would."

Now, if you asked me my philosophy, beliefs about open or closed caskets, I would have said—Closed. Why would anyone want to look at, touch the lifeless remains of a once warm and vital being? You are supposed to remember people in life, not the still unmoving, unseeing, unhearing, unfeeling effigy of who they were. Right? Doesn't that make sense?

But this was the third time I had to face a death and I NEEDED to see each one of them. My dear friend Sheila who died in a car crash the very night she was celebrating her divorce from her sadistic, abusive husband; my Dad ten years before and now my Mom. I had to see her one last time. And truthfully, when I think of her, I think of how she was in life. This was NOT an indelible image that replaced all the waking memories of her. She lives in my mind as the woman she was in life. I can't even remember how she looked in the casket. The one thing my dead mom and live mom had in common—was that "cold" that was so easy for her . . . .

\* \* \*

So there I was, driving down Rt 93 to Plymouth NH having a conversation with Mom and she was answering me, using my vocal cords.

"Mom?"

"Hi Dahlink, how's my Soorala?"

"I'm fine. How are you?"

"Good. Better than I imagined. Everyone is here! It's wery nice."

"Really, mom!? What's nice about it?" (Forever the interviewer)

"Vell, Zadie is here, and Bubbie and Aunt Henchie, and all my cousins who died in the concentration camps, and my grandfather who still lets me comb his beard, and Uncle Bennie. It's vunderful, really."

"That's wonderful Mom. What do you do? How do you spend your time?"

"Time? Dahklink, vat this mean, time?"

"You know, day, night, days, weeks, months?"

"I don't understand, my sweet Soorala. Vat do you ask me?"

"Hmmmm. Well, what happens where you are?"

"Ohhh! Dahlink, it's wery nice. Your fotter and I valk and valk and valk and wisit everybody. It's so vunderful to see everyone!! In fact, Daddy is calling me now. I have to go. Love you Soorala. Call me again, ok? Bye."

\* \* \*

Back to when I was on the cranial sacral table, right after Mom passed, the therapist invited me to see my mother. I think he thought I would get some important loving message from her. I guess I was hoping I would too.

What I saw was Dad who was already on the other side, come to greet her with a big smile on his face. He gently took her by the hand and the two of them walked off towards the light. She never turned back, never looked at me, all I saw was her back. Once again she turned her back on me.

* * *

I wanted to call Jill sooooooo much today, or text. In fact, I've had to resist the impulse to contact her all week. I don't know how I didn't, don't. I keep thinking, if I could just ask her why? Why not talk about it so we can figure it out? How can I make it better?

Or, if I just give her the opportunity to talk she'll open up, tell me what I did to upset her so deeply, how much she misses me too; tell me what a hard time she's been having, but Oh Yeah, these wonderful things happened too. Really wanted to tell me about them but couldn't; she couldn't get herself to reach out to me. Felt embarrassed. Wasn't sure if it would be a good idea or not. Wasn't sure she wanted to put that pressure on herself.

Then she'd be holding back about her other best friends and feel uncomfortable. She'd probably feel overwhelmed and angry with me again, justifying to herself why it's so important to stay away from me. I was too much, wanted too much, expected too much, didn't **really** get her.

Or, more likely, I call her and she's cool, short, says she's about to go somewhere and hangs up.

How could I have felt such intense feelings with her, from her and think that she's not missing me. But she's not missing Stalker girl, right? Right! She was relieved to be rid of her. She's probably relieved to be concentrating on her kids and husband and be rid of me.

I keep talking about my feelings around Jill in my own therapy, in my coaching sessions. But the pain is still here, sometimes dull, sometimes stabbing, sometimes throbbing, sometimes thrumming in my core. Not quite as shocking as the first couple of days, but in some ways more painful. How is it possible?! It's been over 3 months!!! [But who's counting . . . ]

We haven't run into each other. I've had no indication from people we both know that she's mentioned me. But then again, I'm not talking to them about her because I don't want to burden them.

When it first happened, I thought maybe we would figure it out in a few days, a couple of weeks. Even though I was screaming inside—hurt, fury, never again, I can't ever let her hurt me like this again; I still wanted her to come after me. Still wanted to go after her, but she has turned her back on me. Cut me out of her life. Decided that I'm a lunatic to be avoided at all costs . . .

.

# CHAPTER THIRTEEN
## "Love Test"

I know that Jill represents the loss of my Mom, early on. These are very little girl feelings, not self-sufficient grown up Sharon feelings. I'm high functioning; I haven't depended on anyone to take care of me financially ever since I was 11. I've worked hard on my psychopathology so I could have a better life, a meaningful life, a successful marriage. I know lots of people and have many casual friends, people who would like to be closer.

But Jill was different. She was someone I really wanted in my life. I chose her. Like Glenn who I chose for my soul mate.

Out of all the people in the world, I chose him to be my love.

Out of all the people in the world, I chose HER to be my friend.

Why him?

OMG, soooo many reasons:

When I was so enamored with him, and considering letting him deeply into my heart and being, I actually took a love test to see if I was being honest with myself about him. There were 150 questions. I tried very hard to be "objective" in my responses. Really?! Yeah, well . . . Of course he passed with flying colors.

He's gorgeous—just my type, tall, black curly hair, intense black eyes, light skin, little nose, sweet, sweet smile, cushy lips.

He's strong and gentle—He's so big compared to me and solid. I could rest on him without fearing I'd crush him [unlike the little people in my family. I'm 9" taller than my mom and 3" taller than my dad].

He's deliciously seductive—When we were first getting to know each other he used to come up behind me and slip his arms under mine and around my waist. Gave me the chills each time . . . .

He's a talented jazz pianist—he would sit down at piano and improvise with fingers flying. His music was complex, sometimes dark, always intriguing.

He's a learner—has a voracious appetite for information and knowledge across many disciplines.

He's got a vivid imagination.

He's a quick study.

He's introspective.

He wants to do well for the world.

He's a great teacher.

He is charmed by kids and childlike qualities in everyone.

He loves dogs and cats and happy to share our home with them.

He's very entertaining—he took on a project to make me laugh 3x's per day and he's really good at it too!

He's a compassionate listener.

He's a creative problem solver.

He likes to build things.

He's soft over hard muscle.

He's dedicated to health.

He likes to help people.

He has interesting guy friends.

He's a prolific writer.

He lets me know I'm the only girl for him in the world.

Why her?

Her eyes come alive when she's happy to see you.

She's beautiful. I always told her I loved her little upturned nosey [I'm beginning to think I have something about noses. Hmmmm . . . How odd!]

She's smart.

She's imaginative.

She likes to laugh and laughed at my jokes all the time.

She's interested in health and organic eating.

She's a creative cook.

She's a great writer.

She thinks deeply.

She's a good listener.

She expressed interest in me.

She was amazed at my work and so complimentary about it.

She thought I was beautiful.

She thought I was funny.

She thought I was so accomplished.

She thought I was smart.

We were soul sisters.

She seemed to accept me as I was.

Oh well . . . Guess not.

My therapist reminds me that we have less in common than I think. I'm a business woman, traveling, consulting with large corporations and brands. She's a mom of young kids, at home, dealing with the PTA [or whatever they call it these days] and keeping her home organized. We run in different circles.

But that was appealing to me. I haven't lived that life. I have lots of nieces and nephews, but it's not the same. I like kids, like watching them, playing with them. It felt like a perk to our friendship.

More importantly, is that she does not sustain intimate relationships with women. She has that history. The only one she stays connected to is the woman who makes fun of her, connects on a superficial level, is fine with intermittent contact.

Ugh.

But is she thinking about me? Today!? Now!? Do I appear in her dreams too? Am I a representation of unfinished business for her?

I hate this torment, this longing for more torture, this unrelenting need to fix something that can't be fixed.

Face it, Sharon. You are never going to have a Magic Mommy. And, you're never going to have a soul connection with Jill. It's just not going to happen. You were looking through a distorted lens that made her appear like "the one."

So FRIGGIN' sad!!!!!

# CHAPTER FOURTEEN
### "Ache"

I woke up feeling down, a little depressed. Like heaviness that surrounds me. Going through the motions. Seems like so many steps just to get ready to go out the door to get my hot Dunkin Donuts to get my motor revving. Go to the bathroom, brush my teeth, wash my face, put on some moisturizer, grab something to wear, eye drops before contact lenses so I can wear them longer, Vitamin C drink, thyroid supplement, drops for this, drops for that, wait five minutes. Take a couple of other vities. So many steps before I can step out the door with pups in tow. And that's just to get ready to exercise when I get home.

I met a couple of friends for dinner last night. One is leaving to live in CA, opening up a salon and boutique with her sister. The other is in transition too, just differently. Aren't we all in transition? Daily?! Hourly?! Life is transition, right?

But sometimes I want it to stay constant. When you find a pattern you like, that works, why can't it stay just like that? Do this, do this, now that, now this and so nice. So comforting . . . . So satisfying . . . . I hear myself whining inside even though I'm trying to sound normal, grown up.

I was really happy for a while when things were going well with Jill.

Will I be happy again? I feel like I'm floundering. Even though I'm working, doing things, taking care of my little family, writing, there's an ache that I carry. Pain wells up in my chest and flows thickly to the back of my throat, up the back of my head and pushes tears behind my eyes that I blink back.

Why not let them escape?

Seems useless . . . .

What do you want to cry about?

I'm a fully grown woman who feels unfulfilled.

Unfulfilled?

Still sloshing around in the dirty water of my past; I keep trying to clean the floor with a bucket of grey water and no faucet to refresh it.

What do you need?

I don't really know.

What do you want?

I want to make lots of money working from home, without all the travel so I can raise puppies comfortably, knowing I won't have to periodically abandon them.

I want to be thin and strong and soft and hot.

I want to write books about psychic characters with special powers that surprise and delight people, especially me.

I want to LOVE eating totally healthy organic foods and share them with others in a cozy community eating and meeting place.

I want to paint, create, and build a following.

I want to blossom into the interesting, colorful and caring woman I'd love to spend more time with.

I want to remember that things are possible. I want to remember the things that are possible.

I want to create an environment that attracts people I like to be with.

I want to feel complete in myself so that . . .

So that . . . a sob is escaping from my chest in to my throat . . . .

So that, I NEVER NEED ANYONE AGAIN.

SCREAMING, STREAMING, TEEMING, CAREENING

COLLOSAL COLLISION OF FEELING AND MEANING

I hate missing Jill and feeling so powerless about it.

I hate wanting a friend so desperately that I feel almost dysfunctional [although no one else would describe me that way, but no matter how much I go through the motions, it's just that.]

I'm whining and clutching myself, "Why did she leave me?! What's wrong with me?! Why can't I let go of this?"

My therapist says it was an infatuation. Not real. It was chocolate and sugar—nothing substantial, just tasty.

But my feelings of excitement and temporary completion [what an oxymoron!] were real. They were real. I felt them. I experienced them. I knew them. They had valences. Some days higher or lower but always present. I never got tired of her. I never got tired of the feeling of everything was right.

When Glenn and I got together, he said to me, "I'll be your Mommy, your Daddy and your Dog." We laughed and repeated that to each other a number of times when we felt detached from others in our lives.

Why did I not know I was entering a dance that had an end to it? That the music would stop and another piece would start. I wanted to replay it. Pick the best parts and play them again. I want to replay the good parts, but how can I do that knowing how it will end. Because I could reach out to her and probably work it out to have another dance. But it would end again with more torture.

I had dinner last night with two women who are separate from their men. They were talking about how women don't need men. Remember that old feminist saying, "A woman without a man is like a fish without a bicycle."

I never believed that.

Is it a woman without a true friend that's like a fish out of water?

We come alive in the vital, nourishing womb of a loving mother, with hopes and dreams of colors and textures and sensations and experiences and mysteries and problems to solve. That environment of acceptance, appreciation and admiration makes everything possible. I felt so alive and happy in the reflection of Sharon in Jill's eyes. So I guess it makes sense that I feel so dead without her approving mirror. Now when I look I see disdain, darkness and death.

\* \* \*

I want to write something else about it, to lighten that up. But I just don't have it right now. Sorry.

# CHAPTER FIFTEEN
"When Life Gives You a Lemon . . ."

Glenn went hiking today. I wanted to go with him, but had appointments. Took care of stuff, exercised, did some work, procrastinated, went food shopping, met the IT guy to set up my new assistant on her computer and sunk into still another gloomy feeling.

Do you ever watch *The Voice* when the judges are reaching out their hands deciding whether or not to push the button, waiting till the last second and then deciding? I find myself rooting for the performer, "Push it Adam! Push it!" Glenn says I get so involved, that I jump right into the TV as if I'm there.

That's how I felt today driving back and forth from the health food store. I had my finger out poised and ready to push Jill's number.

*Hi Jill.*

Pause. *Uhm . . . Hi?*

*Hi. How are you?*

(And before she has a chance to respond . . . .)

*I just want you to know that even though we're not in contact anymore, I want us to be ok if we run into each other somewhere. So it's not awkward.*

*You know. I don't want to be the coffee shop you can no longer go into because you got your husband to curse at them for making you feel uncomfortable that you left your dog in the car for hours with the windows closed on a hot sunny day. It's a pity you just couldn't say, thanks for being concerned about my dog. Don't know what I was thinking. I'm so glad she's ok. And yes, if she was in trouble I would have wanted you to intervene, even if it meant breaking the window. She's my little girl too. I guess I misjudged the weather.*

*Instead you called Jim, told him how they abused you, humiliated you in public, so he came storming up to be your knight in shining armor and screamed at them, cursed at them with the big F-U, F-U F-U and you have never gone back, even though you LOVED going there.*

*So I don't want to be that in your life; another place to avoid out of fear, embarrassment, remorse. But I flatter myself. And if I do, I apologize. Maybe you just really don't like me, find me disgusting, pathetic, sniveling, whiny, clutchy, desperate; the way I see myself in this mess.*

I'm out of the car in my driveway, pacing, pacing, not knowing what to do with myself.

WHY?!!!! Why did this happen? Why am I soooooo, so upset and stuck?

I start each day with good intentions and then I sink back into the morass.

Uhhmmm. What a weird word morass. More "ass"? What on earth would that mean? I never thought of it that way before. Haaaaa! I can hear you laughing that big laugh. We would have both laughed at that, wouldn't we?!

Like the time you were teaching me to make hummus? Your hummus was so yummy and I'm nowhere near being a cook. You were showing me how to soften up a lemon to get more juice out of it. But what you didn't realize was that they were these huge Meyer's lemons that are already pretty soft. So you started rolling the lemon on my cutting board, leaning into it to give it weight and SPLAT!! The lemon cracked open; a screaming citrus maw.

I seized the opportunity, picked up the lemon and let it speak from the new mouth it had sprouted.

"Oh My Gawwd!" it lamented.

"What were you thinking?!

"Are you crazy?!!

"Damn girl.

"Now look what you've done."

Your eyes opened wide with surprise and mirth, and we both laughed hysterically for several minutes. I can't help but smile writing this. It was one of those ridiculously funny moments you always remember.

It's one of those moments I associate with how much I enjoyed making you laugh.

I have a secret comedienne that lives inside me. I get soooo much pleasure out of making people laugh, particularly getting them on a roll, so that everything you say after the first chortle, keeps getting funnier and funnier even though it's really not. But you've built on the momentum from the previous story so that someone begs, "Stop! Please, I'm going to wet my pants!!!"

My mother, my sister and I used to do that with each other. And I never thought about it before, but I guess that was my doing. I would be the clown, get them laughing, my sister would add something, and we'd be on that roll, laughing so hard that we didn't understand the comments we were making because they sounded like gibberish. And then he said, blah, blah, blah blah, Haaaa! [Squealing together] AND that was funny in itself. So we laughed harder and harder till Mom usually had to run to the bathroom and Penni and I caught our breath.

Jill, I always have so many things I want to tell you—annoying stuff that happened, touching things that I know would touch you, always the funny things, realizations about things that seemed to come out of thin air. It's sooooo sad to me that you're not there. But even worse to think that I was so awful that you had to totally cut off from me! [I see you rolling your eyes. "Not that you were awful, but you were too needy; wanted too much; wanted to own me and I won't be owned by anybody. Do you hear me!?! No one, no matter what! Now leave me alone!"]

I'm still having a temper tantrum with myself about this. Nooooooo!!!! This can't be. It was just a thimble! Why are you giving me the silent treatment? And now you're dead and totally silent. How can that be?! I can't accept it. I don't want to accept it. You were a mediocre mother at best, really a pretty crummy mother to little Sharon, but as long as you were alive there always seemed like there was some hope to work it out.

As long as Jill is still here, maybe I can work it out with her.

But I know I'm kidding myself. Just going round and round, wishing for something that is not possible with her. It wasn't possible with my mom. Maybe it's not possible with anyone.

# CHAPTER SIXTEEN
"Letting Go"

I want. I want. I want . . . Feel empty. Unfulfilled . . . foggy . . . . Want to go back to sleep. But I'm not tired and have too much energy to stay down.

I read a quote by Maya Angelou on the day she passed. It reverberated deeply . . .

"I don't know if I continue even today, always liking myself. But what I learned to do many years ago was to forgive myself. It is very important for every human being to forgive herself or himself because if you live, you will make mistakes—it is inevitable. But once you do and you see the mistake, then you forgive yourself and say, 'well, if I'd known better I'd have done better,' that's all. So you say to people who you think you may have injured, 'I'm sorry,' and then you say to yourself, 'I'm sorry.' If we all hold on to the mistake, we can't see our own glory in the mirror because we have the mistake between our faces and the mirror; we can't see what we're capable of being. You can ask forgiveness of others, but in the end the real forgiveness is in one's own self." Maya Angelou

Can I forgive myself for losing Jill?

Can I forgive myself for wanting more than people can give in return? At least the people I choose? There are others who can give as much, I'm sure, but I don't find them. I don't recognize them. How can I when I continue to look for the familiar? The original love in my life . . . ? That was painful to write. But what did I know?

I was an infant, a baby, a toddler, a child who had real needs. I was dependent on her to keep me alive. Not able to do for myself. But now I can. I do. And yet, I spiral over that original sin, original pain, original loss that gets repeated, repeated, repeated, endlessly, a whirlpool in force, pulling me down. I'm being dragged down by the weight of the swirling water. I hear the rushing, the raging sound, spinning faster and faster until, I'm lost. I can't hear or see or feel . . . anything.

It's like Tommy.

"Hello . . . ? Hello . . . ? Hey . . . ? Can you hear me . . . ? Do you need a hand?"

I groggily open my eyes. What the heck? Did I pass out?

What am I doing? Where am I? On a big wet grey slab of rock deep in a giant hole in the ground. How did I get here? I'm cold and stiff.

"Hey? Do you need a hand?" There's someone up above looking down. A guy in a work shirt and jeans!

"Is this your dog?"

I see Stewie, my Shih Tzu looking down, panting, tongue hanging out, whining a little, doing that little bowing dance that Shih Tzu's do.

"I found him sniffing in the tall grass and he ran over here. That's how I found you. You OK? Do you need a hand? You look like you must be freezing."

I tried to sit up. I was sooooo stiff, muscles tight and achey. How on earth was I going to get out of here?

"Yes. Yes I do need a hand."

But I was afraid to let go, to let go of my hold on the cold slab. Was afraid to sit up . . . . I hadn't even looked around to see what was beyond the rock. Was there a deeper hole I could fall into? Would the whirlpool return?

"It's ok." He called. "I have a rope and can throw it down to you."

"You have a rope? Why do you have a rope? Are we in Texas?"

"No need for sarcasm, Ma'am. I can help you out. You'll be fine. Just let me throw you this rope and help you out of there. Ok?"

What choice do I have?

"OK" I yelled back up. "But I'm afraid to let go."

"You'll be fine. I'm going to make a loop and lower it down. Once it's near you, all you have to do is bring it down over your head to your waist. Then hold on to the rope and I'll pull you up nice and slow."

"You really do sound like a cowboy. What are you doin' in these here parts?"

"Ma'am?"

"Sorry."

He lowered the rope, very slowly. When it got close to me, I braced myself with my left hand and reached out to the rope with my right. As I did, I could see the edge of the rock and realized that there was water below, like some giant well beneath me. I felt woozy.

"Go on now," he said gently.

"I'm feeling a little dizzy, afraid I may slip."

"You're fine. Just take that rope and get it around you."

Ok. Ok. I take it gingerly and pull it over my head. But Wait!! What if he's a psycho and is going to pull it so it grabs me around the neck and hangs me!!! I forget my dizziness and quickly pull the loop down my body, anchor my right hand so I can slip it under my left arm and panting yell back up.

"It's around my waist."

"Good. Now keep it a little slack, grabbing the rope with both hands and I'll start drawing you up."

Oh my god, what kind of crazy movie is this?!

I feel the tension on the rope and it starts drawing me up. My heart is pounding, afraid my hands will slip. Now I'm standing and soon on tippy toes.

"Let your feet hit the sides of the walls and try to push up against it, a little, ok? Like you're climbing up"

"Ok," I answer nervously, not knowing if he can hear me, but unable to allow my voice out any louder.

The rope is pulling and my body is swaying. Are my arms strong enough to hold me? All of my strength is in my legs. So yes it would be good to be pushing at the chunky earth walls with my feet. My foot grazes the side. I try to gain purchase but my foot slips, the dirt is slimy and kind of smelly, rotten egg-ish. Makes me not want to breathe. I feel that awful sense of falling even though I'm still holding on for dear life.

"Good. Push down again," he calls to me. "It will help us get you up, faster."

I feel myself scrambling against the wall sometimes making contact and often just flailing. But I can tell that I'm on the rise, coming out of my 6 feet deep.

I can see the surface, Stewie's little face watching me, panting, the stranger pulling on the rope, hand over hand. I feel the air, warmer and sweet smelling, I can see the sky, slightly overcast but clear. A ridiculous thought goes through my mind, "are there tics here? Am I being saved only to get Lyme disease?"

Did you ever notice ridiculous thoughts in your head, almost as if someone else was saying them and shock yourself that it was you who thought them? I've had a number of those moments. It's like catching a glimpse of your-self unexpectedly in a mirror and seeing yourself the way others see you.

One classic example was a time Glenn and I went to the movies. I needed to use the rest room afterwards. So I walked in and saw several people standing at the sinks and heard myself say to myself, "What a bunch of ugly women!" It took me a second or two to realize I had walked into the "Men's" room. With a jolt, I went running out, shocked at how my brain had processed seeing men when I was expecting women. It was a funny, but not so nice thought.

So here I am trying to escape this sink hole. My arms are so tired but I keep a tight grip until I'm just about at the top and he reaches down to take my hands and pull me up the last couple of feet.

I'm on the grass. It's fresh and warm and softer than the cold rock. Stewie is all over me licking my face. Can't help but smile at him even though I'm scratched, and everything hurts. The man asks permission to remove the rope from around my body. I raise my arms and allow him to take it off me.

"You ok?" He looks at me scanning my eyes for a real answer.

I think to myself. Clearly I'm not ok or I wouldn't have been swallowed up by this, this, this what?

A whirlpool!? Hole in the ground!? This can't be real. Where am I anyway?

I look around and see my old office in the background.

I remember a few years ago when Stewie ran off into the tall grass behind the old house that was my office. Couldn't believe he ran away. I chased after him, calling him. He didn't respond. I saw a path in the midst of a stand of tall grass. A man came sauntering out of the grass holding Stewie. He looked just like this guy. Tall, slim, in jeans and a plaid shirt, dirty blonde longish hair, blue eyes, gentle smile. "Is this who you were looking for?" he had asked.

"Yes! Thanks. He ran off. Thanks so much for catching him!"

"No problem. He's a cute little guy". Then he nodded at me, turned around, and disappeared back into the tall grass.

Wah? Where did he go? Where did he come from? At that time, I just scooped up Stewie and headed back to my office to tell the people in my office about this mysterious stranger.

And now, here he is again. I don't know how I got here. I was feeling down and swept up in my discomfort and then find myself in a hole . . . well I already told you that part. I thought it was my imagination, but here I am in the grass.

Again, he asks, "So are you OK?" "Is there something you need?" "Can I help?"

OMG, is there some THING I need? I need soooo MANY things, sooo much. How can I answer that? Is my car here? Do I have to walk home? Where are my shoes? What time is it? Where's Glenn?

Where is my friend?

"Uhm." Looking down, a little embarrassed, ". . . I just need to find my sneakers and Stewie's leash. I just live a couple of miles away. I, uh, I can walk home."

I look up and see my sneakers and the leash and . . . no cowboy . . . again. I come out of my reverie, my waking dream, because I wasn't really asleep, just sitting here kind of meditating and then there I was.

So weird! I had incorporated a real memory into my imagination. That really did happen a couple of years ago with the stranger coming out of the tall grass with Stewie, turning him over, smiling, and then vanishing into the grass. So weird! And so interesting that I used him to save me from my living grave!

# CHAPTER SEVENTEEN
## "Guilt is like Cancer"

Jill, I had a very satisfying, incredible day of coaching! I want to tell you all about it!!! It was exciting, exhilarating, healing, nurturing . . . I feel sooooo full of these people and their important challenges.

Is it just the "E" in me that wants to be seen and affirmed by someone I like and respect? Someone that has nothing to gain or lose by giving me feedback . . . . Why can't I just look in the mirror and tell myself, "Girl, you did mighty-good! Not bad for a white girl!" I hear Dahlia's deep, mellifluous voice, "Girl, you give so much of yourself. That was amazing. Thank you. Thank you. Thank you. God bless. You are . . . ."

I am what? What do I need to hear to heal the wound that lives deep in my heart?

One of the women in our coaching program was stricken with colon cancer, Stage 3. I was afraid to talk to her, hold her, would I absorb her pain and, as an empath, feel and live her challenge? Could I rise to the occasion?

She came to my/our Group Coaching class today. I saw her name and felt . . . scared, worried, uncomfortable, checking out my body for possible problems—like a scanner going down my body looking for problems, Meeeeem, meeeeem, meeeeem, white light, yellow light, purple light, white, yellow, pink, green, yellow, pink, blue, deeeeep blue like deep water. All is fine. Phewwww! I'm ok.

I want HER to be ok. She's so inspiring. Helps people get over their addictions, keeps a sense of humor, works hard to learn, change, be present. And SHE has colon cancer? WTF? How can that be? I can hardly bare it.

AND she's the first one on the class call today. What do I say? What should I do? Tell her how crushed I feel that she, of all people, could be smitten with this horrible affliction. Cancer!? Colon?! She has a 9 year old little boy! I thought only old people were affected. This is wrong, ridiculous, WRONG!!!!!

If I let myself think about it too much I could get swept into a panic. I have to stay calm and focused and sound normal so she doesn't feel my internal frenzy.

"Hi! How are you and I'm so glad to see you here."

She responds in her normal voice that always has a bit of a laugh hiding behind it.

"Hi Sharon, thanks for all your well wishes and I'm glad to be here."

Other people join in. Caring well wishes are expressed. Then the conversation continues as usual. Topic changes to the coaching issues at hand. Everything seems back to normal.

What did I expect?

I expected my long suffering mother to make me feel guilty and indebted to her, "You owe me for letting you live. I could have taken the ergot but I didn't. I suffered to keep you alive. I should have let Daddy get rid of you. My life would have been easier, better. I liked being the only woman and then you came along. It was better before with the three boys. I didn't have to worry about them becoming whores. It doesn't matter if boys are naughty. Well maybe it does. Look what happened with your brother. How dare he? Comes home and tells me he knocked up a girl. 17 yrs. old? Was he crazy? What else could I do? Told him to marry her right away! And that family! What a bunch of crazy people, white trash."

"Mom . . . ! Stop . . . !" I hear myself screaming in my head. "It's bad enough you forced him to marry her. We don't even know if it was his child. Stop it. He's not bad. Well he wasn't bad back then. He needed help. He was lost, didn't know what to do."

"Why did he have to tell me? He should have taken care of it. He was making money. I wouldn't have known the difference. He should have kept it to himself instead of making me the laughing stock of the family. Ooooo, Tillie, so high an' mighty but has a son and daughter in law who are . . . tsch tsch tsch."

"Mom, nobody cared one way or the other. But you made poor Jake miserable. He had an awful life; always the outcast, always miserable. He died of a broken heart Mom. As soon as you died, he followed you to the grave. All he wanted was you."

"Yeah, well he's not here. Thank God. He must have gone to the other place where he belongs. Toi. I'm through with him."

"Who else are you through with Mom?"

"Will I ever be through wanting you to really be my Mom?"

# CHAPTER EIGHTEEN
"Addictions"


But it was soooooo much fun to have a soul sister.

I misjudged her. I thought she was capable of being my friend forever. I thought I was capable of being her friend forever.

STOP IT! JUST STOP IT. Enough already! Move on. It's time to move on.

Comfort food—starchy, heavy, fatty, pleasing to the palate but overly filling—makes you sleepy so you can rest, BUT makes you F-A-T!!! Just not worth it, my sugary soul sister. I had a teacher once who talked about Carbohydrate Men and how women were attracted to them. How they were addictive and wreaked havoc on their systems.

I did gain weight being friends with Jill. She cajoled me to eat sweets with her. She stayed slim but I started to gain weight. Did I do that to protect her? To let her be the sexier one?! To avoid competing so she wouldn't feel threatened? Or did I just enjoy the indulgence and want a place to blame for my lack of discipline? Eating too much sweet; sugar is addictive. Starch is addictive. Jill was an addiction to me.

What's the nature of addiction/people addictions?

It always starts out great, chemical, chemistry, magnetic, magical. Feels so good, you've gotta have more. Every bite, sip, encounter is soooo delicious— like sugar, alcohol, drugs.

Yep. That was what it felt like. Even though I didn't pursue the friendship for several years, each time I saw her there was that eye widening, big welcoming smile, a kind of knowing/recognition as if we had known each other for years even though we hadn't spoken for more than a couple of minutes. I felt happy seeing her . . . like a little sparkle light had danced into my day.

There's a primitive type of reflection and joining. *"This is the only friend who ever understood me."*

And I did feel like that and so did she—or at least that was what she told me over and over.

"You really get me! It's like we're thinking and feeling the same thoughts all the time."

We merged like mother and newborn in those moments; One person instead of two. True love that nature grants to the mom so that the baby will be cared for until she's ready to go out on her own, feed herself, and fend for herself. My mother wanted me to believe that she was the only one who loved me, understood me—BUT she really didn't understand many parts of me. As I began to differentiate and become my own person, she became more and more controlling, forcing me to be like her, do like her, feel like her and whenever I didn't she would withdraw so I would feel the pain of losing her attention. I'd be pulled back into the drama, terrified of being abandoned. The more I tried to grow the less she gave and the more she pulled away, or hurled insults. "You're just like your father!"—Overly emotional, out of control, tragically flawed, male . . . BAD!!!!

Maybe Mom might have seen me for who I was, if she hadn't cut herself off from the feelings that she judged as bad, socially unacceptable. Instead she acted on them, pretending that she had all good intent. Soooooo many times putting out, pushing the poisoned apple to squelch me, to stop herself from seeing me as separate.

Addictions invite overindulgence, dependence and abuse. The user ends up feeling sick from the substance and worse if she goes into withdrawal. And addictive relationships and substance abuse do not endure change and growth. It gets more and more intense until something cracks, breaks, dies of an overdose.

# CHAPTER NINETEEN
"Boy am I Bugged"

It's been 5 days since I've sat down to write.

What a weird way to start. Is this a confessional? Who's the priest? Why do I feel kind of guilty? Like I was not being responsible by going about my life, working very hard, not even having time to exercise and getting minimal sleep, traveling from city to city to city, dealing with difficult people, solving recruiting problems, handling cranky people in the backroom, holding their feelings so they can sit back there and listen as cooperatively as possible . . . AND yet here I am I starting my day feeling guilty that I haven't done enough.

Ok. Ok. Just observe it and move on. You're not going to solve a problem of a lifetime in one writing post.

As rigorous as this week was, I really did enjoy learning about people who were devoted to their cats.

I spoke to people in four cities around the country to find out how they felt about their kitties and the foods they fed them. The kind of work I do gets to the underlying feelings people have about a given life situation, problem, available solutions and imaginations about the ideal solution.

The types of things I've studied are numerous ranging from more obvious things that someone trained in psychology would be invited to study like depression, anxiety, bipolar disorder, drug addiction, diets, etc. to diseases and conditions such as cardio-vascular disease, hypertension, Parkinson's, Alzheimer's, MS, cancer to lighter things like toys for tots, bottled water, protein bars, skin care products, eye drops, yogurt, cookies and now Cat Food.

I had everyone introduce themselves as their cat. If they had more than one, I asked them to pick their favorite one. No one balked. Even though they ALL described these little critters as a child to which they were "Mommy" or "Daddy" [in their own unsolicited words] and it would not be PC to say you have a favorite child, they were readily forthcoming in selecting their special kitty and instantly transforming themselves into Spooky, Smokey, Peanut, Taz, Ghetto Boy, Sweeto, Sturgis, Catzilla, Purrfect or Ramone for their intro.

When big, burly 40 something Jason channeled Ramone he appeared with a charming, seductive hybrid French/Euro accent that sounded just a bit like Count Dracula.

"So nice to meet you, Sha-rone. Thank you for having me. I am Ra-mone. I loooovvve my humans. They are so good to me. They took me off the streets when I was a scared, defensive, and as you say, 'scrappy' teenager and gave me the family I never had. They plied me with tasty temptations and healed my wounds— outside and inside. They let me sleep with them and cuddle, pet me, let me entertain them. It's just delish. I'm soooooo lucky to live with them"

A couple of cat people demonstrated their cats' aloofness. When I said Hi, they turned their heads and pretended to look somewhere else.

Almost all changed their voices to a higher pitched lilt that mimicked a meow. At times I felt like I really was talking to a cat.

More than anything, kitties brought them joy, comfort and calm. No matter what kind of chaos was challenging them, the presence of this playful, energetic, soft, comforting yet comic character enabled them to get back to basics, what was real and truly important to them, to relax and de-stress and stop taking the problems in their lives too seriously. It was a return to innocence, to the simple things that made life meaningful.

I've had a cat since I was nine, well up until we moved to NH. We rented for the first year. Unfortunately, the home owner had a thing against cats, while dogs were fine. So we found homes for Fred and Wilma, which left us feeling guilty, sad, lonely for them, but it had to be. Stewie and Zach were allowed. People are sooooo weird. Cats are very clean. Why would anyone object?! Dunno.

The weirdest thing was what happened when we moved out.

Right before we found our house, there was a fire in the house we rented. I was out of town, Glenn was at a meeting, the housekeeper was doing the laundry. She turned on the dryer and POOF, POW, the damn thing went up in flames! Apparently they hadn't serviced the dryer in 10 years. There was an accumulation of lint in the whatchamacallit, where it wasn't supposed to be and POOOOF! Electrical fire!

Tanya, ran out of the house cell phone in hand and called 911. It happened so fast that there was a lot of damage. We had to move into a Sheraton while they were making repairs.

I was in a high travel period. After spending the weekend with Glenn and the pups, I left for a 5 day stint on Long Island. That had a nice benefit of allowing me to see my old hair dresser.

Jocelyn washed my hair and began blow drying when she commented, "What's happening, Sharon? I've never seen you have so much dandruff . . .

"Uhmmmm . . ." her usually soft, mellow voice transformed to a high squeak. "That's not dandruff . . . That's lice!!!" Looking at me—my face, which was stretching into a shriek; my hands reaching up to my head then stopping in the air to avoid touching my hair—Jocelyn reclaimed her cool as I started to freak out. She excused herself, called her husband and told him to bring her a box of Nix immediately.

I was a little out of my mind as you can imagine. It didn't occur to me to find out what was in Nix. Glenn and I are health food junkies and try to avoid as many non-organic products as possible. But LICE?!?!?! Whatever it takes. I itch even now, any time I think of it.

Back in command, she assumed her nurse persona, assuring me all was fine, we'd take care of everything right away. She Nixed my head, made me take off my clothes, jump into a shower and gave me something to wear. God bless this woman!

I was shaken. We played detective and tried to problem solve how this might have happened. After some serious investigation, and talking with the Long Island hotel I was staying in, it became clear that the offending space must have been the NH hotel we were camping out in while the fire damage was being cleaned up. That meant I had to call Glenn and tell him to get himself checked out.

Of course, no one wanted to inspect his head. He had to go to 3 hair salons before anyone was willing to examine his hair. Yeeeeesh!

AND, fortunately, he was clear.

Hmmmmm. Then I remembered. On Sunday night, as we were relaxing and watching TV, I was cold. I pulled a blankie out of the closet and wrapped it around my head and body, sitting in a chair, looking at tv.

The blanket?!?

That was the only difference.

OMG!

We had to tell the hotel. We had to fumigate our clothes, everything. Cost a fortune. Ugh. But what's money compared to LICE!!!

Did you know that lice prefer a clean head of hair. Oily hair is not appealing to them. But the typical person would think that Lice means dirty person, right?!

I was soooooo shocked, ashamed, uncomfortable in my self. How could I walk around, be with people in any personal way knowing I'd had these critters in my hair, on my head. AND, I ITCHED!!!!!! For a whole month afterwards. Every night, I made Glenn check my scalp. Ugh! What a horror.

It made me remember being in 2nd grade and finally having a friend, Laurel. She was a bit of a waif, but she sat next to me and I liked her. I invited her back to my home after school one day. My grandmother forced me to sit with my head under her skirt as we played in the enclosed front sun porch.

"Gramma, Stop!!!"

But she wouldn't.

After Laurel left, Gramma admonished me for bringing home this dirty girl with bugs. Wah? I had no idea what she was talking about. I liked my friend. My grandmother always blew things out of proportion. Did she see bugs? No. She saw a child who could have been wearing nicer clothes and have her hair combed. That was all.

But, I have to say that after that my feelings about this little girl changed. She became "dirty" in my mind. Unfair? Yes, totally. But I was 7 and highly impressionable.

One day shortly after the visit, Laurel threw up in her hands in class. Ooooooooo, yuch. Everyone gasped and expressed some utterance of revulsion. That was it. I was convinced that she was indeed dirty. And definitely smelly. Gave up on her as a friend. Sad.

BUT, OMG, how must I be with head lice?!!

Gross, disgusting, a leper who could affect/poison others. What a creepy feeling.

And the hotel? What did they do? Gave me credits towards another stay after blasting the room with toxic chemicals. Yeah, right. I'm really going to stay there again.

HAAA! Just noticed my email. I received an invitation from Starwood Preferred to update my password. The universe has a sense of humor, doesn't it!

# CHAPTER TWENTY
## "Mother Love"

We went to see Maleficent last night. Glenn was humoring me because I allowed him to take me to Godzilla a couple of weeks ago. I dunno. Watching giant robotic monsters mechanically duke it out just never did anything for me. Glenn, on the other hand, was super pumped watching Godzilla vomit raging energy into Mothra's mouth, frying him from the inside out. Must be something to do with testosterone . . . . Last night, looking at the movie marquis he actually suggested we see it again. Uhm, maybe next week?

Maleficent was very touching and surprisingly meaningful to me.

Brought up so many questions:

- What defines a woman?
- Is she still a full person if she doesn't have a man as the love of her life? Does Maleficent ever

SHARON LIVINGSTON, Ph. D.

get to have adult sexual interactions with anyone?

- Is the love of a mother truer than the love of another?
- Is mother-love just the representation of self-love? Or is it what allows self-love?
- Is there such a thing as true love from a significant other?
- What is more enticing than sexual love? Enough to tempt betrayal of the love object?
- How much does power corrupt? And what does it take to heal corruption? To heal Betrayal!?
- What is the ultimate betrayal?

Here I go back to Jill. I felt betrayed. I had given myself over to her as much as I could with any friend and she rejected me. Ouch!!!!!! Ouch, ouch, ouch! How could she, blah blah blah . . . I've already told you that part over and over.

But the bigger betrayal is to me. I betrayed my own trust in myself by choosing, yet again, someone who would help me replay the excruciating feelings with my mother.

Judgments, humiliation, self-doubt. Down, down, down girl! Don't peek out from behind those false beliefs. Don't let your true self show, because she'll destroy you—destroy the spark, destroy the curiosity, the creativity, the joy of discovery and experimentation, destroy anything that might take way from her being the woman in the family with the men's full attention on her.

Can I ever forgive myself (or Will I ever be able to forgive myself):

- For cruelty I've shown myself?
- For the lack of understanding of my own needs?
- For getting (being) blind-sided?
- For doing this to myself?
- For shutting myself down, and (unwittingly) trying to obscure my own light?

I forgive you Sharon.

I'm soooo sorry you went through all this without me by your side, helping you see the truth. But we were soooooo little. No way could we have known. You needed her back then to survive.

It was awful that she left you time after time and terrified you with threats and horrifying stories. She wanted you to think she was magical and if only you did the exact right thing, gave her exactly what she requested in her puzzle spell would you have her love and . . . acceptance? Admiration!? [Right? Really! Forget it]

Be the only child she truly wanted? Or, if you were magical enough, powerful enough to cast the exact right spell, then you could change all of the hurt she felt so that she could emerge as a complete person, full of caring and capability to give love to her little girl. But you were too strong to totally submerge and drown, become her zombie. And you were not the magic she wanted.

# CHAPTER TWENTY-ONE
## "Dreamscape"

### Dream

I'm at a local gathering place where a workshop is about to happen. Coffee Shop? Village Bean? Something like that. One of our mutual friends is presenting on meditation or something like that. I see Jill over to the right. I feel very awkward. We catch eyes, dull eyes, indifferent eyes, as if I'm not really there. Well, you're not! It's a dream! There's no connection, just recognition of a shell of a memory. I look away.

# CHAPTER TWENTY TWO
## "Dependency Revisited"

So here I am still torturing myself about torturing myself. I know you get it. I'm OCD, stuck in a rut of replaying the same old tune. Everyday I go over it over and over and over again. I go over "it?"

What's the IT? Is Jill IT? Is Mom IT? Is the hole in my soul, IT?

IT is gnawing, annoying, poking at me, pointing at me, making me question my neediness, my obsessiveness, my worth as a human being. How can I help others when I have IT haunting me, taunting me, relentless. Is IT my companion? Never leaves me alone? Even Stewie doesn't stay by my side all of the time. But IT seems to.

Maybe I just need a constant companion because I can't see myself without one. Like contact lenses for my inner vision. But sometimes lenses distort. They maximize or minimize trying to bring sight into reality and balance. Maybe I've minimized the importance of early pain for so long that I need to maximize now to finally see it for what it was? To finally let go of expectations?!

I'll never be a baby again, a toddler, a child, not even a teen? I'll never get the needed unconditional care from a mother. How can I? I'm an adult and have been grown up for many years.

Stalker. I still have that word stalking me, punishing me. Could I really be a stalker? I've helped others who were dealing with others who were hooked on them. I know what stalkers do. Am I really a stalker and just lying to myself? Hmmmm.

I go back to an old file that I put together for a client to help her figure out what was happening with an old boyfriend—although the same behaviors hold true outside of love sex relationships.

Do I do any of this with Jill?

- You are being stalked when someone persistently watches, follows or harasses you, creating fear or insecurity. No
- A stalker can be someone you know, a past boyfriend or girlfriend or a stranger. Yes

A stalker may . . .
- Follow you, hiding from view. No

- Come to your house, office without an invitation. No
- Constantly, test, call, leave messages, send you letters. No
- Send stuff—gifts, flowers, weird stuff. No
- Call and hang up. No
- Try following you and tracking what you're up to on social. No
- Spread rumors about you in your community or online. No
- Park at places you might be seen. No
- Become friends with your friends to find out more about you—in your community, on facebook. No

Phewww! I'm not a Stalker!!!! Yay!

Well yeah, there are some aspects of stalking that I have not mentioned here. In my mind I think about her everyday. I think of my Mom every day, too. Am I stalking my dead mother? Is it stalking to want to process something? To work it out of my system?!

What will I do with my time when I'm not obsessed with Jill anymore? What did I used to think about before she was there to fill the space that exists here? What space is that?

What does it take for me to detach from pain? To let myself heal?! I keep reminding myself, going over events, wondering what I could have done differently to avoid the toxic attachment. Because it was not healthy for my system as evidenced by this treatise to pain, right?

# CHAPTER TWENTY-THREE
## "Just Whistle"

You're not going to believe this.

Have to give you a little background . . .

So, I haven't told you this but my husband is very sensitive to sounds. Extraneous or loud or shrill sounds distract him and rattle him to his core. I have something similar to that. I have a high startle response with someone "appearing" when I don't expect to see anyone. So Glenn has learned to make a soft sound when he's padding into a room in bare feet so I realize he's there.

AND, generally I avoid distracting him with sounds. But we both do forget at times when we're caught up with something else.

Hmmmmmm. It just occurred to me . . . . I'm a highly visual person and he's highly auditory, so I guess it makes sense that it's an unexpected visual cue for me and an unexpected auditory cue for him that goes into sensory overload. Actually never thought of it like that before. Very Cool!

So, the other night, we were getting into the car to go to our favorite organic restaurant for dinner. It was still cool enough for the pups to come along. Stewie jumped in but Zach was procrastinating. Sometimes he needs some encouragement even though he loves joining us and hates being left by himself. Sitting in the front passenger seat of Glenn's Odyssey, and forgetting about Glenn's sound sensitivity, I turned in the direction of the open van door on the driver's side and whistled. Glenn yelped and shot me a stricken and angry look. My first response was defensive, mirroring back his annoyance with my own unintentional but deadly glare.

The thoughts that went through my head were something like, "well if he had just gotten out of the car and went over to get Zach, I wouldn't have had to whistle! It's his dog, why can't he take care of him. Why do I always have to jump in and help out. Geeeeez!!!" As you can tell, I'm not so great at holding back my facial expressions of my feelings even though I'm good at not saying them out loud. Ugh.

I can't remember exactly what he said but it was voiced displeasure at both my high pitched whistle in his ear as well as my defensive denial of it. "I just wanted to help you get Zachie in the car" is what I said when he expressed his irritation.

That response, coupled with some negative expression on his face further fueled his displeasure. So both of us were frustrated and upset with each other and both of our feelings were hurt. I wondered whether we should abandon our dinner plans because it would be 40 minutes in the car. Could we drop the uncomfortable feelings and have a nice dinner? I knew my hubby was looking forward to it.

By this time, Zach had hopped into the car and Stewie had settled himself on my lap. I took a breath, quieted myself and changed the subject, asking him about his day. We both breathed more comfortably and headed for the highway.

Dinner was nice. While waiting for our kale and tempeh to appear, we were able to snuggle a little on the cushioned bench seat that we liked to share. Life seemed good again. I really LOVE talking with my husband about our program and goals and how we are doing to get there. It's fun, exciting, stimulating to figure things out.

We independently discuss our lives with our own coach and mentor. He's been very supportive of what we've created. And he does support journaling about our lives. That's part of how I started this treatise on loss.

Recently I had told him about thinking about publishing what I had written as a book. He basically told me not to.

Wha? Uhm, why not?

I felt devastated because this was the most creative thing I had done in a long time. I've been feeling so alive—getting up several times per week and putting my thoughts, feelings and imagery down on paper— well a paper looking screen.

I really felt crushed and depressed. What was I missing? Why did he want me to stop? Was I being to mean to Jill? Should I not be writing about real events? Rather than feeling outraged, I pushed down my anger about it/denied my feelings and just stopped writing. Instead of waking up with excitement about continuing my story, I moped through my mornings before getting to work and turning my attention to the "important" things, not my recreational writing.

So when we were getting out of the car and coming back into the house after our make-up dinner, Glenn told me that he had had a discussion with our coach about my "book," this that I am writing now.

He told the coach that it was powerful, expressive, creative and entertaining. He thought the sentiments and insights would be helpful to others' growth AND that he believed we could publish it easily. He said more that I don't recall exactly because I was caught up in an incredible wave of peace and admiration.

Myyyyyyy heroooooo! I was swooning. You stood up for me? Reallllllllyyyy!? OMG! I was just about flabbergasted. Really?! That's what you told him, that you couldn't wait to hear the next installment? I almost sat down on the floor, unable to contain my joy. I've always longed for a protector but have been so busy being strong and safeguarding others that I don't inspire that urge, even though I greatly crave it.

It meant so much to me that my husband appreciated what I was writing. He's always thought that my articles on research and branding were well done, but this was different. I've been revealing the real me in raw form. And to have him like it, love it, and want to have me share it with the world, because it would help people unravel their own thoughts and feelings about the events in their lives . . . was . . . was . . . astounding? Touched me to my core? A soft, thick comfortable blanket I could relax into? The best hug I had ever felt in my life? Safe, supported, sustained, and seen by the most important person in my life. It was a moment I wanted to remember and cherish forever.

And then he said, "That's the Sharon I married." And that was the beginning of the end of my inner peace. My suspiciousness coiled up. I got very uncomfortable, but said nothing for about half an hour. Then as we were getting into bed, I could no longer contain my discomfort and invited the pain. You know like asking your husband, well how fat do you actually think I am?

I asked him sweetly, "So how am I different from the Sharon you married?" I hear impending shark music in my mind, but persisted. He says, "Well, you know, this is so sweet and vulnerable and funny and insightful."

"And I don't seem like that ordinarily?"

He pauses.

"How am I different?" I'm thinking, hey, this is the real Sharon. I'm so much healthier and more vulnerable than I was when we first met. What the heck [actually had nastier words in my mind, more like WTF] are you talking about?

He said, "Well I was thinking. You know that part where you talk about your Dad throwing down the cartons of eggs . . ."?

"Yeah . . ."

"I was thinking that it's kind of like that."

Now I have *Psycho* music shrieking through my head as Bates is approaching the shower but not sure who is Bates and who is the victim in the shower.

OMG! He sees me like my crazy, anger management candidate Father? The one who beat me?

More *Psycho* music . . . .

"Ohhhh," I say hesitantly and pull off to my side of the bed.

All I can hear in my head is my mother's voice, "You're just like your father! You're just like your father! You're just like your father! You're just like your father." It echoes in my mind over and over as I try to breathe, remember that my husband really does love me and try to calm myself to sleep. Not the time to talk. I'll get myself in major trouble with both of us.

I'm crying inside. This is such a repeat of my past. I would get warm and vulnerable with Mom and she would take that opportunity to teach me a lesson, a lesson that would hurt to my core twisting as it made its deep scarring impression. Crying now . . . hotly, but quietly.

# CHAPTER TWENTY-FOUR
## "WTF!"

Next day . . . . Wake up . . . . Had a rough night . . . .
Try to be friendly to hubby even though I have the
echo of Mom's voice still there. I remind myself that
Glenn is not my mother, and that I've lived with him
longer than I did with her, that we have a great
relationship but all relationships have painful moments.
That I need to find out what he really meant about me
and my father and to avoid exaggerating and making it
bigger than it is.

I have lots of work to do, interviews with Kitty
owners via InterVu a fancy Adobe Connect webcam
system that allows the clients to watch remotely as I talk
to the participant also on the internet, showing them
materials, using a white board to draw and enter text.
Very cool program that I'm excited to do. I know

Glenn and I will work this out and that I have to attend to my project.

Day starts off with some minor glitches and then we're on a roll. The system is easy and the clients are thrilled being able to watch and interact with me behind the scenes. It's seamless and I'm delighted that everything is running smoothly including drawing Cat Chow packages with my track pad. The kitties I attempt to draw via the cat owners instructions are a little weird, but identifiable as felines.

Every now and then I check my email to make sure all is in order when I see this, the note below . . . from Jill with the subject heading, "sent to wrong address: *I think I sent this to the wrong email address so I wanted to send it along again. Sorry if you are receiving twice*

*"Hi Sharon,*

*I hope this message finds you great, happy and healthy! This note has been on my mind and in my heart for a while now and I thought it the right time to share it with you. I apologize for it being an email however I'm much clearer in my communication lots of times in written word, thank you for the indulgence of that. I've wanted to let you know that I'm grateful for the time we shared a friendship and sisterhood. For whatever reason that I'm not able to understand and probably don't even need to at this point, there were some challenges that we weren't able to overcome. It's okay for BOTH of us. I can speak for myself in that I learned a lot about love, life and growth, personally, during our shared time. I have absolutely zero hard feelings for what happened. It has not been easy by any stretch of the imagination and I have run the gamut of emotions as a result of what happened. I have peace now and know that it's all okay. I have had probably the biggest "growth spurt" of my life since January. I have lost relationships and have shifted and although it's right it hasn't always been easy. I want you to know that I have nothing but love for you, Glenn, Stewie and Zachie. I know we tend to show up at things at the same time, our parallel worlds :D and I want you to know that when we see each other again, I hold nothing but love for you. Truly from the bottom of my heart.*

*Thank you for the love, lessons and gifts that you brought to my life!"*

AHHHHHHHH!!!!!

What the hell?

Are you kidding me?! That's what I wanted to write back?! Are you friggin' kidding me?

I could hardly get myself back to work and I had 3 more hour long interviews to conduct, all friendly and inviting and open and responsive and listening and attentive and . . .

I'm feeling out of my mind with, with, with . . . energy sparking, spitting, flying about.

OK, calm down, calm down. It's ok. You can think about this later . . . call me Scarlet O'Hara . . . I forwarded it to Glenn, well maybe this can be a peace offering too and went back to hearing about the cute kitties and their capers.

# CHAPTER TWENTY-FIVE
"Remembering Dad"

It's Father's Day.

So?

Yeah. I'm supposed to remember my father, my father who wanted me dead. My father, who my mother hated and loved; My father who screamed at me, beat me, ignored me most of the time; My father who loved my little sister but thought I was a pain in the butt. Did he even know I was there? One time, after I dyed my hair red and started juicing with lots of carrots, he came to visit with mom, saw the carrots going into the juicer and said, "So that's what happened to your hair!" He occasionally did have a sense of humor.

After he died, Mom used to speak to him in the middle of the night when she was lonely and couldn't sleep. She would look up to the ceiling, because she was in her bedroom and could only see the ceiling, but imagined she was looking into the ether realms, and say . . .

"Samilah, dahlink, how are you? I miss you. Dahlink, vat are you doink?"

She was never good at ng's or w's.

"Samilah, I can't sleep, tell me dahlink, vat should I do? I'm so tired but I kent sleep?"

She told me that he told her to have a little schnapps. And so that's what she did.

What gifts did I get/might have gotten from my father?

My creativity, love of art, smarts, generosity, ability to teach, humbleness, shyness, intense feelings, passion, silliness, and ability to attach to another AND . . . a belief that men were intense, scary and explosive or dark and retreating into their own inward torture chambers. Holding all his jealousy, judgments until they were too much and erupted.

My father ADORED my mother. He was smitten the moment he met her.

They were first cousins, but they didn't meet until she came to this country at the age of 16. He was 14. They were both very shy, but being cousins they were thrown together. He felt responsible to help her assimilate to the US culture. She spoke no English, only 6 European languages. The first time he met her, he invited her to go for a walk, motioning to her. He reached out his hand holding a piece of fruit and said, "peach?" It happened to sound like "vagina" in her native tongue. She blushed deeply and they were off to the races. He pursued her valiantly for 5 years until she finally said, "Yes."

This included following her when she went on dates with other guys and literally pushing one of them off the bus so he could spend time with her. He claimed chaperon privileges since he was her cousin and they were not worthy. Ha!

She finally succumbed. She had been deeply in love with another Sam, a lawyer who was destined to be very successful. One day, in a fit of anger he broke up with her, broke their engagement and instantly married another woman. My mother was shocked and heart broken. She loved him and did not understand why this had happened, but was appalled that he turned to another. He annulled the wedding and came back pleading forgiveness, but Mom was having none of it. When my father showed up on her door step she told him she would marry him. It happened very fast; a small wedding in a beautiful dress crafted by my grandmother. And, well, they did have 5 kids, so I guess in the end my Dad's approach was successful.

# CHAPTER TWENTY-SIX
## "Torture"

I did not respond to Jill's email. It's been 5 days.

I sent it to Glenn, read it to my mentor, shared it with my writing coaches. I feel guilty knowing on some level I'm torturing her back by my silence.

But what's the point of responding?

What good will come out of it?

She's self-centered and unwilling to look at what happened; to work through what it might represent, how it might be healed. She said she had losses, plural. She's had many losses in the short time I've known her. She's ended a whole series of different kinds of relationships because the other had done her wrong in some way.

She is not interested in hearing my thoughts. She just wants to put an end to it BUT be social when we happen to meet accidentally in our community. So she can be comfortable and not have her moment tarnished by Sharon, one of her many stalkers.

It is clear to me that she assumes we will be showing up at the same places like we always have in the past. Maybe she has been avoiding going places where we often ran into each other—the yoga studio, a party given by a mutual acquaintance, Whole Foods where I shop twice a week, one of several coffee shops and lunch hang outs we both like to visit?

Am I cruel in allowing her to continue worrying, and not spare her the discomfort? How many other people has she hurt with her lack of awareness? With her tacky mesh of emotional entrapment. I'm feeling outrage instead of guilt right now. Oooops. Here comes the guilt. Ugh.

Ugh.

I say to myself, she's doing the best she can. That's all she has at this moment in time. Maybe in ten years she'll be different? It's not as if she hasn't thought about it, but has not been able to figure it out.

No hard feelings? Really?! What did I do to you that engendered hard feelings? Ask you if you were OK? *Son of a bitch!*

Sorry for swearing, but I'm infuriated all over again. OK, it's my responsibility for texting her, expecting/wanting to connect daily even though she said she wanted that kind of connection . . . . Oh stop it, already.

She has hard feelings about what she perceives you did that she's denying. AND you know she denies lots of her feelings, projects them out so others feel them for her. Then she separates from them because they are too uncomfortable. I represent her wanting and neediness.

Does she represent how much I reject myself?

Sharon, honey, it's time to embrace yourself, to be your own woman, your own person, regardless of how others see you. You are a good person, a person with a full range of feelings. You were gifted with intensity. It gets you in trouble sometimes, like now, but also works soooooo well for you when you're in your creative process, when you're problem solving a complicated research issue; when you connect with others and feel their feelings so they can relax; express and move on to solve another life puzzle.

Remember, there will be lots more puzzles for you to consider. There will be more people who need you and hopefully are open to being needed too.

Let's learn from this experience and read the signs early so you can touch the surface, feel the lure, the heat, the ache, and make a conscious decision to walk away no matter how tantalizing the drug.

Can you do that? Can we do that?

Dunno. [Just call me Harry Potter.]

I know that when I work out gently over time, my muscles get stronger. Sometimes when I push myself too hard I have temporary setbacks from injuries, mostly minor. Once I was out of commission for 4 months with intense sciatic pain. I did a series of stupid things that really hurt me; things I knew were ridiculous, but I was trying to be Super-girl. [Isn't it interesting to note that Jill and I became friends just when I was finally getting over that injury!? Hmmmmm. Have to think about that.]

So if I can take my time, be nice to myself about how I got caught up with Jill . . . If I give myself my observing ego to look for me when I see a yummy looking cupcake with incredible creamy chocolate frosting . . . If I invite my mind to protect my heart without closing down . . . If I can be my own best friend, taking little Sharon by the hand and having our own special adventures and talks . . .

I'm optimistic. That is a part of me that lives on always, even when I'm disappointed.

I got over my sciatica, when lots of people do not. I do my 100 flights of stairs every day. I CAN exercise heart wisdom going forward.

# CHAPTER TWENTY-SEVEN

What is it about 5 days? It's been 5 days of lower back pain. I've been to the chiropractor 3 times, saw the acupuncture gal yesterday who saved me four years ago, and this morning my back hurts more than it has all along. And there's some numbness going down my right leg. It's freaking me out because I remember the 4 months of pain and numbness that made me feel ancient, incapable, frustrated and frightened.

This is minor. I'll get over it. I probably shouldn't have done my 100 flights on Monday, two days ago.

What if my L4/L5/S1, lower back could talk?

"Slow down. I'm going to make you slow down."

"Why?"

"I need some attention."

"What do you want?" [Sounding annoyed]

"You just expect me to jump without gently loving me and helping me wake up."

"Ohhh, you're not a person, you're just a set of bones and ligaments and tendons and muscles"

"Right, and I need to be warmed up before you use me so intensely. I need to be handled like you love me. You just put all this pressure on me and never give me time to recover. So I'm enforcing recovery time now"

I went for a therapeutic massage two days ago. FINALLY, relief! And you know what she told me? Apply heat before you exercise. You need to warm up the area to avoid irritating it. Really?! My talking butt knew the answer all along?

# PART TWO

Revival

# CHAPTER TWENTY-EIGHT

So the passion I have writing about the Sharon and Jill saga is cooling down, just like my previously inflamed lower back. Can I write without upset? Without pain?

Strum, strum, strum . . . . Clicky noises on the keys but no words coming . . . . Hmmmmm.

Well, what have I learned through this process?

Lesson One:
Eventually the pain subsides.

Jill is retreating into the distance. Her face is becoming blurred; the bright eyes harder to see. I dreamed I ran into her at a public venue. This time there was no change in my pulse. We acknowledged each other, nodded with tiny smiles and looked away.

The doom and gloom are lightening. I wake up thinking about what the day has in store for me. Before getting her "love" filled email, I woke up daily thinking about Jill. Whyyyyy?!!!! What's wrong with meeeeee?!!!! How could she not want me anymore?????

And then I'd answer myself.

Well . . . .

You're too intense.

You want too much.

You lose your boundaries when you love.

You impose yourself like a cute 3 three old, hopping into the lap of the other thinking, somewhere actually believing you're still little, adorable, funny, full of life that is contagious and they're ready and big enough to hold you and play with you, be entertained and keep you entertained.

You are still looking for a complimentary mirror in the eyes of a mother/playmate, affirming, validating, and appreciating. It's as if you don't exist but in the reflection.

You're just tooooooo hungry. You don't know how to eat in small doses. There's no internal monitor telling you when you've eaten enough until you're too full and the object has been fully consumed, till there's nothing left.

Wait a second. This is NOT an inanimate object that I devoured, even if I wanted to. Jill was living and breathing and athletic. She could have asked for limits, but she didn't. I should have recognized her limits, but caught up in the replay of child needs, caught up in my own narcissism; I saw a beautiful mirror and was trapped in the beautiful likeness, seeing myself in her admiring eyes.

When the eyes closed, I felt lost, worthless, condemning of myself and the mirror. There was no Windex to clean it. It just was fogged over, smudged, with spots that could not be removed.

I felt like I could hardly live without it. Now that I had found this magical mirror and lost it, how could I see myself so positively?

When the fog cleared, I saw different realities.

A greyed, old, mean image, an ugly, evil old witch, trapped in darkness, wanting revenge, wanting to destroy.

A dirty little orphan in tattered rags, tear streaked face like painted lines through the grime; huddled in a corner of a street, wondering what would become of her and expecting nothing.

A 5 year old having a temper tantrum, kicking, screaming, and crying tears of rage, hard to get close to without getting hurt.

A sickly woman lying in bed, ashen, drawn, and clutching her chest silently imploring God, "Why hast thou forsaken me?"

Mom!? Is that you again?! Ugh, pulling myself out of this self-effacing but negatively gratifying set of reveries.

I see myself jumping into a hot shower with Oribe shampoo and conditioner that smells so good and is so refreshing and hydrating to hair, a bergamot soap from Whole Foods that also excites my senses. I let the hot water sting my back and cleanse my body while the mixed bouquet of fragrances lifts my spirits so I can start again.

This time when I clear the fog off the mirror I see myself as grown up Sharon casually walking down a country road. I see a little girl sitting under a tree, looking dejected. As I get closer I realize it's me.

I'm at first, surprised, and then very interested to get to know her/me a little better, so I say, "Hi, how are you today?" She looks up with a sad face and returns her gaze to the ground where she's playing with a smooth stone.

"Phew, I'm a little tired from my walk. Mind if I sit here with you for a couple of minutes?" She glances at me suspiciously for a moment, but when she sees my unflagging smile she nods her curly little head.

She nods at me again, indicating it's ok for me to join her. I watch what she's doing, drawing squiggly lines in the dirt with her stone. I ask her what her name is. She draws it in the dirt.

S H A R O N

I say, "Wow!!!! That's my name too!!!" She looks up as if to say, "Really?!" I nod and smile, "Yes. And I spell it just like that." I ask her what she likes to do. She shrugs her shoulders and looks down continuing to trace lines in the dirt.

"Do you like colors?" Her face lights up just a little bit as she slowly bobs her head up and down, three small nods. I reach into my satchel which magically appears. It's relatively small but there seems to be limitless space and items inside. I explore the contents until I find what I want and pull out a large sketch pad and a box of beautiful soft sticks of pastels.

I ask her if she'd like to play with them. She's a little hesitant but then extends her hand into the metal box and pulls out a rod of a rich, deep red.

She opens the drawing pad and looks at it as if not knowing what to do. I tell her, "Go ahead, it's all good, whatever you do. Art is limitless. It's whatever you'd like to express. It's fun. Try it!" smiling at her encouragingly.

She draws a light thin line with the edge of the pastel. Then she presses down a little more firmly and the line thickens as it angles down and then turns and begins to trail up the left side of the page before it stops close to the top and heads back to the right. She draws two arches adjoining on top. As I continue to watch I realize she's drawing a heart with a hard line through it.

She looks up at me with what appears simultaneously to be a sad, yet hopeful glance and then draws her gaze back down holding the stick of color poised above the paper.

"It's ok." I say to her. "It's a beautiful little heart. What lovely arches it has."

She touches the soft color on the page and notices that it smudges easily. She takes the pastel and adds more color in the middle of the heart and then uses two fingers to spread it. The heart is filling with the hue in varying shades as she smooths it around. It's beginning to seem fuller and textured. Hey, she's only five but able to image a 3D looking heart. How cool is that!

"Good!" I say with some exuberance in my tone, but I try to keep my enthusiasm in check, so not to scare her.

She glances back up at me, acknowledging me with one of her little nods, and then continues her work. She adds a lavender layer that gives the heart more dimension. Then she takes a pink pastel and draws lines emanating from the heart center. She smudges them so they look like gentle rays of sweetness radiating.

"Come On!" I think to myself, "this little girl knows about heart Chakra" But I stop my critical self, hoping it's not showing on my overly expressive face and return to focusing on her instead of me.

Her face has become flushed. She's drawing and smudging faster. She fills in the background with beautiful blues and greens and purples. They start to encompass the heart, so she brings back the reds and pinks so it looks almost as if it's pulsing with energy.

I look at her and see that she is covered in pastels— her hands, her clothes, and her face where she wiped her hair away with her pastel clad hands. Now she looks a little like that street urchin, but this one seems happy and involved. The sharp red line that originally penetrated the heart is almost invisible, like a pale scar—there but almost imperceptible.

I tell her, "Wow, that's beautiful!!!" She smiles shyly, then points to the purple. "Mommy doesn't like when I like purple."

"Really? Why?" She shrugs, her little hands facing palm up, pouting lower lip, knit brows over wide eyes.

"Who doesn't love purple?" I ask in astonishment. "It's beautiful, rich color that's magical and royal."

She shrugs again, shooting me a quizzical look.

"I'm not allowed to wear purple" she mutters under her breath.

"What honey?"

A little louder, "I can't wear a purple dress or pants or shirt or hair bow!"

"Really? Does she tell you why?"

She hesitates as if she is not supposed to tell me. Then she whispers, "She says shvartzes wear purple."

Whaaaat????

And then I remember. The color purple. Not the work of Alice Walker, but the prejudice held by my striving mother who was trying to prove that we were not the same kind of poor as the women of color who were my nannies and housekeepers. So odd!

My usually generous mother looked down on Black people. I cringe to say that out loud. We were not

187

allowed to eat out of the same dishes even though they were allowed to prepare my food. Whah??? How can that make any sense?

Mom came to the US with virtually nothing and lived in low scale housing until she married Dad. They lived a humble life for many years, Dad working as an insurance salesman in a black territory while Mom brought up my 3 brothers and helped my Grandma run her store in South Jersey. Dad got sick and could no longer make the house calls for his district. He quit the insurance business, laid up with some weird form of eczema that was debilitating. Both he and my mother blamed his malady on the conditions that his poor black customers lived in and endured.

Mom could cook up a storm. Dad convinced her to cook for a store of their own. He knew the Deli business because he helped his parents in their store. Mom's creations were better than Grandma's. So Mom prepared the food for the new Deli and womaned the counter while Dad did the books and back room operations—ordering, finding bargains, checking inventory, supervising the cleaning, hiring. They finally started making money after I was born.

I was raised by Katherine, my black nanny who dressed with flourishes of color and probably lots of purple. I adored Katherine. She was fun, would take me on outings, to her apartment, dress me up, feed me . . . And then one day, Katherine was gone. I was very tiny, just 2-1/2 or so, but I remember missing her and feeling devastated that she had left.

My brothers told my mother that Katherine showed them her breasts to get them to do things she asked. My mother believed that Katherine was meeting her boyfriend at her apartment for afternoon delights with me in the other room. My mother also believed that I was beginning to love Katherine more than I loved her . . . , you get the picture. No more Katherine; Heartbroken Sharon.

I never had a nanny again. My mother tried to replace her with 'nice' white nannies but as the story goes I threw a tantrum every time someone was introduced to me. I do remember one of them. I saw this woman walking up the stairs towards me with wild blonde hair, green eyes and a long nose with a wart on it. I screamed at the top of my lungs at this witch coming to eat me and that was that.

I think I unconsciously was trying to keep Katherine with me with my love of purple and distaste for my mother's prejudice. I would ask about her incessantly at first and then from time to time over the years. Mom was always defaming her character in one way or another. I never got to see her again, was not even allowed to know her last name so I might find her myself one day as a grown up and thank her for saving my little life.

I look at little Sharon and say, "Wait, I have a surprise for you. What's your favorite thing to wear this time of the year?" She shrugs but looks at me expectantly. "Do you like to wear dresses? Pants? Shorts? A top and skirt?" She sees me rifling through my bag, gets up on her knees, puts her little hand on my shoulder and tries to peer inside. "Underpants" she says with a little mischievous grin on her face.

I say, "And, what do you like to wear over your underpants?"

"Overpants!" She giggles.

"OK, enough joking, really, what would you like to wear today?"

She thinks for a minute and says, "A ballerina dress!"

"Great," I say, still searching, not knowing what might really come out this magical bag, and then I find it—a cute little purple tutu with lavender chiffon and fairy sparkles all over it.

"How about this?" I ask holding out the dress. Her little eyes broaden and sparkle, her face cracks into a huge smile, and she tentatively takes the tutu in her hands.

"Can I wear it?" she asks hesitantly

"Of course you can. The magic bag made it just for you!"

I'm thinking to myself, "Hmmmm, what other magic is hiding in this bag. I wonder if it's got a sweet purple Mercedes SL 500 sports car in there."

# CHAPTER TWENTY-NINE
## "Intense"

It's 5 days again and I've been revisiting Lesson One from time to time this week, feeling . . . well it's hard to describe. I couldn't believe that I started with a simple statement reiterating that "time heals all wounds" and lapsed into another reverie. I thought I was going to be concise. Can't stop a rambling mind, I guess.

Lesson Two:
Find your flaw and see the strength in it

As I thought about what I contributed to the demise of my relationship with Jill, I realized that from her eyes I must have appeared hungry, consuming, constantly in her face, possessive, you know, the Stalker.

I was not able to control my wanting enough, even though she has no idea of how much I was holding back. I wanted to tell her everything like a little kid who's learning to talk, experience, comprehend and sees the world as a magnificent delight of forms, colors, sounds, textures, feelings, puzzle pieces that are beginning to fit together into a 3D painting. That was my narcissism. Wanting a magic mommy to accept me and love me for my innocence in inhaling the world. I quickly learned that I was supposed to listen to her issues without judgment, empathize, say "Awwwweee, THOSE BASTARDS! No wonder you feel that way!" Just like I learned by age 3 that to get my mother to engage I had to ask her to tell me stories about her when she was little. And that worked with Jill, until the BASTARD was me, of course.

I was a BASTARD because:

- I challenged her boundaries.
- I invited her to consider her part in the bad things that were happening to her in her other relationships. I did that without suggesting it, but just letting her talk had to open the door for questions about why all these awful things were occurring over and over with different people.
- I wanted to claim her as my best friend. She said she wanted a best friend and there I was, ready and willing. But in her mind, that needed to rationalize why she could never have a best friend although she desperately searched for one, I was not able to be there for her.

- I was just too intense with all my feelings.

Shame looms in my core, like a heat that travels up my abdomen to my stomach, to my chest, to my face that colors with humiliation. I was too much. I wanted too much.

You know the joke about the guy who goes to see the psychologist. The psychologist says, so what brings you here today? The guy says, Doc I keep vacillating. I'm a tee pee I 'm a wigwam, I'm a tee pee I'm a wigwam, over and over in my mind, I'm a tee pee, I'm a wigwam.

The psychologist looks at him and says, "Ahhhl, I see the problem, you're just too tense."

Dreams are like that sometimes. When there's something we are almost ready to hear from our depths it comes up in the form of a pun or a weird image or kinesthetic cue. If you say it out loud to yourself or write about it and reread it, or tell someone else, a different perspective can reveal the true meaning that was hiding in the code.

I've been told I'm too intense at various times throughout my life. It was a criticism. I've worked on myself in serious psychotherapy, coaching, studying psychology, behavior and I remain "intense" although I try to contain it. I think being intense is a part of being Sharon.

What does intense mean?—According to Dictionary.com: "of extreme force, degree, or strength; e.g., the job demands intense concentration" or" having or showing strong feelings or opinions; extremely earnest or serious. E.g., an intense young woman, passionate about her art."

Synonyms for intense:

- Passionate/Impassioned
- Overpowering
- Serious
- Ardent
- Fervent
- Zealous
- Vehement
- Fiery
- Emotional
- Earnest
- Eager
- Animated
- Spirited
- Vigorous
- Energetic
- Committed
- Fanatical
- Extreme
- Great
- Acute
- Fierce

- Severe
- Exceptional
- Extraordinary
- Harsh
- Strong
- Powerful
- Potent

Hmmmmm. I love some of these!!! [There I go being intense, as in animated and energetic.] Not all of them. Being overpowering, fierce and severe could definitely be disturbing to others and if I want good relationships with people, a best friend, I need to temper those aspects.

But, what if I could focus on the positive aspects of being intense? What if my intensity is one of the "gifts" that comes with being Sharon rather than a tragic flaw?

I thought deeply about this as an intense person would and decided to reframe my understanding. In talking about my insight with John, my accountability coach, I came up with a mantra to give to myself. It's posted on the computer armoire next to my desk.

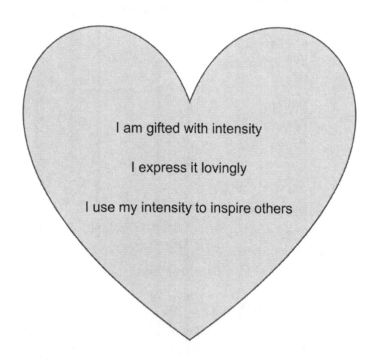

It's a heart. Looks like this.

During a small supervision session yesterday, I shared my heart concept with the two people I was coaching. I invited them to create their own statements while we on our little webinar. I put them into hearts and sent them to each of them.

They both were delighted with their "valentines" to themselves.

I use my intensity to inspire others to reframe their greatest flaws into their greatest strengths. Amen!

# CHAPTER THIRTY
## "Imaginary Friend?"

It's been an intense week. I haven't written in 6 days. At least I broke my 5 day pattern. Always good to do something different, isn't it?

But, here I am again, wondering what I'm going to write about. Do I have something to say?

Strum, strum, strum, and . . . strum.

I sit here at the computer, mind drifting. Trying not to think about all the work I have to do today, finishing my report on Cat Food. Some cat owners actually believe that cats SHOULD eat corn, when it's just filler. Yeeeesh. Just because it's farm grown doesn't mean it's fit for kitties. Can you imagine a lion doing typewriter teeth on an ear of corn?! I don't think so. The king of the jungle is a carnivore and so are all the other felines in our multidimensional jungles. The only time you'll find your cat eating grass is when [s]he wants to throw up a hairball or something that upset its system.

As I sit there shaking my head, I feel a tap on my shoulder. Even before I turn to see who it is, I know it's a man. A Man!? Yow! What is some man doing in my office? I know it's not Glenn. He's upstairs running a webinar. How could a man be here!!

I turn slowly and sure enough I see a tall man with long dark hair in a dark suit with a long jacket, waist coat, legs apart, arms crossed in front on him, chin tucked, standing there looking at me with a kind of amused but condescending smirk on his face, one eyebrow slightly lifted.

So you would think that the first thing that would go through my mind would be What the HELL!?

Tell him to get out. Scream at him to get out! But instead, all I can think of is . . ."OMG, did I comb my hair? Did he see me doing something weird—like scratching under my arm or that weird thing I do when I'm thinking without writing—pushing my nose down to my upper lip. It's an old habit that I try not to do because Glenn thinks it looks weird. One time he asked me, "What are you doing? Are you kissing your nose?" I said, "Of course not!" Then glibly asserted, "I'm smelling my lip!" Made him laugh, but that was his way of saying he didn't find the gesture very appealing so I only do it in private now. But I wasn't private!!

It was another one of those instant associations that seem crazy when you look back at them. Like the time I was hijacked to Cuba. No kidding, I really was hijacked to Cuba in the late 80's. Was on my way to run focus groups on Mellow Roast coffee in Tampa . . . . The flight was taking a very long time, over lots of water. At one point I got up to use the lavatory but was shunted up to the first class WC because someone was being "sick" in the coach rest room.

Turns out that the guy who was being sick was hijacking the plane! However, poor thing was anxious about doing it. He was sitting on the commode with a Molotov cocktail in one hand and a lighter in the other having a panic attack and intense diarrhea . . . .

OMG! How embarrassing! I've been there myself, panicking about something and having to go on anyway. It's humiliating. But . . . You know? Now that I'm thinking about it, how did he get his pants down to use the toilet without fumbling with his bottle of gasoline? And what about toilet paper?! Yuck. Wonder what kind of reception stinky guy got when he greeted his family later that day.

There I go interrupting myself again.

So we finally landed to see a bunch of Russian planes on the side of the runway and when we came to a stop we were surrounded by many men with machine guns pointed at the plane. I could hardly breathe. Talk about panic.

The captain drawled a sarcastic announcement that I think was supposed to calm us down, "Hi Folks. Welcome to beautiful Havana. Apparently one of our guests wanted to come here instead of Tampa. So here we are. We'll be back with you in just a sec."

The plane was totally hushed, every one looking around, checking each other out.

Then a young female flight attendant got on the loud speaker and in a high pitched anxious voice told us that we would be refueling and would get back in the air, back to the US very shortly. Then within seconds, she got back on and loudly squawked at us, "Everybody must deplane from the rear of the aircraft and you must remove all of your personal belongings before deplaning."

Huhhhhh?! They want us to take off our clothes??!!! Barbarians!!!! Now I'm in total shock. I look to my right and see the man across the aisle adjusting his belt buckle. I think I'm going to faint. I mean I had never fainted before, but if anything was going to do it, this would. And all I could think about, be horrified about, was that all of the people on the plane would get to see my fat!!! I must have turned stark white, because the man next to me, put his hand on my shoulder and said, "its ok. Everything is going to be all right." OMG! Did he know what I was thinking? I took a halting breath and noticed that people were getting up and taking their bags with them. Ohhhhhhh. Ohhh, OK, I get it, BRING all your stuff with you.

But that's what I mean. Here's this man in my office, and all I'm thinking about is what kind of impression I'm making. Was I sitting up straight? Did I make any disgusting noises? Hey, it's my office. I don't have to be ladylike all of the time, do I? I wasn't expecting anyone. Glenn would be down later, so I didn't have to be the cute girl while I was working solo, did I?

And then I find myself telling myself, "You knowwww, it's probably a good idea to look good, feel good just for yourself, right? This is about you, not about how others see you. You need confidence that stems from taking great care of yourself, being the woman you want to be, right? Sit tall, look nice for yourself, be the person you want to be. If you think disgusting noises are unpleasant, then don't make them, especially in front of yourself!" I'm thinking, "Yeah, yeah. You're right. It would be good practice to pay attention to my posture and practice how I want to be my best me."

But meanwhile there's this strange person behind me in my office, being incredibly patient as I go through this scene swapping. Patient? Why am I calling him patient? He shouldn't be here at all. So if I'm going to free associate he'll just have to wait!

OK. Sharon, be in the present. See who he is and find out what's going on.

"Who are you?" I ask with a scowl.

He laughs.

"Does it matter who I am? I'm here in your office."

"Well, uh, what are you doing here in my office?"

"Watching you; you're pretty entertaining you know. All of that stuff about how you look and act when no one is observing; very amusing. And were you really hijacked on an airplane? Quite amusing, I must say!" He chortle to himself.

You can hear my thoughts?!!! I'm thinking, in shock.

He cocks his head and continues smiling.

I think I should be feeling frightened, but for some reason I'm not. Just very curious! Who is he? How did he sneak up on me without me knowing he was here? The only thing going is the dryer, which is pretty quiet. I should have heard him. And why didn't Stewie bark? Where is Stewie, anyway?! What does he want from me? Why does he look like he stepped out of a Victorian novel or True Blood?

"How is your dog?" he asks still with that slightly condescending smirk.

What kind of accent is that? One second it sounds Euro, the next almost Texan . . . Texan? Dog? Cowboy???

"Wait a second," I say. "Are you . . . ?" I look closer and notice the same facial features, green eyes, and lean looking frame as the guy who rescued me from the hole in the ground.

A ridiculous question comes to my lips, "What happened to your dirty blonde hair and plaid shirt?"

"You like this look better." He answers.

"What?"

"I've seen all the vampire and werewolf stories you read and you made it quite clear that you are a bit contemptuous of . . . cowboys." "And you unearthed that picture of your man with his long black hair and put it on your desk."

I notice that Stewie is sitting at Count Dracula's feet. When did that happen? Just a minute ago, Stewie wasn't around. He's panting his happy little pant, as if he just had a fun romp or had been 'killing' one of his stuffed animals.

I feel myself becoming highly indignant. "What do you mean you've seen all of the characters I read about? And even if you did, why would you bother? Why would you care? And if you do, why on earth would you show up in my world as a cowboy? [Did I really ask him that? This is totally ludicrous] Why are you stalking me?!!! Who am I to you? What do you want from me? I want you to know right now that I'm happily married and if that's what you're interested in, you need to find yourself another girl."

He laughed out loud. "You are safe with me, little one. We are of the same fiber. We do not mate with each other. We are linked in purpose."

Little one!? Is he kidding? No one has ever called me Little One. I'm the tallest person in my family, taller than my brothers, sister, Mom and Dad.

Stewie was now lying next to the guy, one paw on his boot, gently snoring. That sound usually comforts me. Means he's feeling peaceful and calm which allows me to relax and sometimes actually puts me to sleep. But it's unnerving to have him so tranquil at this stranger's feet. And he was indeed strange. And, PURPOSE? What purpose?

I wake up mumbling purpose to myself.

Was I dreaming? Did I fall asleep sitting in front of my computer? My neck is stiff from being stretched as my head dropped forward chin to chest. Stewie is snoring at my feet, his warm little head tickling my ankle with each breath. Really?! I fell asleep at the computer, sitting in my chair. I shake my head, roll my shoulders and then look behind me. No one there; It was a dream.

I look up at the Word file. I'm supposed to be writing Lesson 3.

# CHAPTER THIRTY-ONE
## "Addictions"


Lesson Three:
Sometimes relationships ARE an addiction

The intense positive feelings we have when we meet someone we think is the love or our life or our best friend are the same ones that are present with drugs. We experience a powerful high from the release of dopamine, the happy neurotransmitter. Being with that person gives you a hit. When people connect with that instant recognition and desire to want to spend time with the other, there's serious blood chemistry that comes into play. During those times people report feeling healthier than usual, being productive, energetic, and needing less sleep . . . .

AND, unfortunately, just like someone recovering from drug addiction, there is a very uncomfortable

SHARON LIVINGSTON, Ph. D.

withdrawal effect until the body readjusts to normal levels of dopamine, serotonin and epinephrine.

These can include loss of appetite, nausea, chills, trouble sleeping—too little or too much, restlessness, nervousness, irritability, anxiety and depression.

But the good news is that we DO recover. The levels do go back to normal. The depression does lift as long as we avoid the substance long enough to let reality return.

One day I woke up and realized I was not depressed. The heaviness had disappeared, evaporated. I felt light, positive, interested in seeing the sunrise, the blue skies, the beautiful spring greenery with it's delicate new leaves. It was such a relief. I woke up smiling and ready like I used to do, no longer dragging and obsessed.

There is a difference in friendships and love relationships that continue in a healthy way vs. those that burst into flame and then just as suddenly die out.

The addictive relationship is all about how I feel when I'm with the other. My sense of self is dependent on the type of contact or lack of contact with the other. A real friendship is about the "we."

When things are not going perfectly well, you remember that you are on the same team. The friendship provides a safety net to discuss and figure things out in a way that protects both of you.

Real Friendship begins with two people who already experience themselves as lovable in at least some ways, rather than being so dependent on the other for validation. You complement each other's strengths and help balance the weaknesses, understanding that sometimes will be harder than others. It's important to remember that we all revert back to childhood wounds that get expressed in the present, even though they originate in the deep past. These are challenges that can help us grow. Rather than being addicted to an ongoing state of bliss in the twinship, we recognize differences and value them.

A good friendship is a place to grow safely, with support and acceptance and trust. AND, it takes commitment and work.

Glenn and I have that. The chemistry was very alluring in the beginning. He was sooooo handsome. Just my type. I couldn't stop looking at him. Truthfully, the first time I saw him, that was all I saw. Big gorgeous guy who left me breathless, stuttering, backing out of the room for fear of embarrassing myself. I had NEVER felt like that with anyone ever before.

I knew enough about instant attraction to know it was alluring, but might be a repeat of something that looked tasty but could be bad for me. AND, I had a boyfriend. He was dating someone regularly too.

So, because we were in a program together we went slowly, getting to know each other over time—in classes, running into each other at the gym or cafeteria, beginning to hang out as friends, talking on the phone.

W both had other love interests when we first met. We'd talk about them. Share, commiserate. Even though there was a strong attraction, neither of us talked about it. We put it on hold and in the process got to know each other.

We started to understand each other—what our hot buttons were, both good and uncomfortable, so we knew how to encourage and also what to avoid. When we finally decided that this was more than a friendship, the chemistry did ignite again but there was healthy protein and veggies under the delicious sauce that made it seem so enticing. So many years later, we continue to be a work in process. It continues to be an adventure that I love. No matter what, we're there for each other, figuring things out, strengthening our connection—laughing for comic relief.

# CHAPTER THIRTY-TWO

Lesson Four:
"Trust Your Instincts"

I knew early on that Jill and I would get into trouble. At that point I could have gracefully pulled back and bowed out. But I thought I was bigger. I'm trained in psychology, for God's sake! I understand her struggle. I've been there. I can handle this. I've got it.

But I didn't have it. I was too quick to react to the tantalizingly delicious rich box of milk chocolates with tiny pits of crunchy almonds in them. Most times I can resist, but I had been exercising hard, working on myself, feeling strong and healthy. What harm could a little crunchy chocolate do? I'll just get back on the treadmill and work it off.

You have to know that I've sworn off sugar. AND starch. They are virtually non-existent in my diet.

[Well, except for an occasional cheat, and I do mean occasional, maybe once every six months?] I'm very sensitive to them both. My body reacts creating candida [yuck,yeast!] which then wreaks havoc on everything. The yeast organisms actually affect your brain because they thrive on sugar to stay alive. Yeast cells send signals to your brain to eat sugar. You crave it; feel like you can't exist without it, while at the same time, feeling worse and worse.

Yeast [or Candida, as it is known in medical circles] can make you:

- anxious
- impulsive
- obsessive, compulsive
- depressed
- have brain fog
- have difficulty concentrating
- feel bad in your body in general and sometimes nauseous and chronically exhausted

I had almost all of those reactions in "detoxing" from Jill. And the detox would start if I hadn't heard from her in just a couple of days. I got anxious. It was hard to control my cravings for her, wanting to phone or text. When I didn't get any communication from her, I'd start feeling mopey. I'd have difficulty concentrating and feel lethargic and foggy. My decision making process was faltering. I felt like I couldn't trust my instincts. That's what addiction does. It breaks the natural machinery in our bodies to know what we know. It destroys our natural instincts.

The lesson here is that we have to be attuned to our instincts from the START; especially in areas that we know we are vulnerable. The minute I had that instant attraction to Jill, I should have been monitoring myself and asking myself some critical questions.

- Hmmm. Interesting. I had an immediate attraction to this person.
- What is drawing me to this person?
- What do we have in common?
- What do we not share?
- How easy will it be for me to have limited contact until I know much more about her?
- What signs of disconnect or trouble are popping us as we do start to get to know each other?
- How easy is it to extricate myself, pull back?
- How often am I seeking contact?
- How rewarding is this friendship? Be very specific
- What is not so great? Be honest

So, what did I notice?
- Intense, sparkly eyes
- Warm, engaging smile
- Felt like I had known her forever—Bamp . . . Bamp . . . Bamp . . . Bamp . . . —sirens should

211

be going off right about now. What? How could you know her forever? You just met her. This is possible projection. No. Not possible projection, but absolutely projection. All you see are sparkly eyes and a nice smile and you're captured? This is chocolate. Buyer Beware! You're in danger of a very rocky road. Back off. Back off. Back off. Intruder alert. Intruder alert. Your heart is in danger of being broken. Take cover until you hear the all-clear siren.

- Who does this person remind me of in any way? If Mom comes up, be afraid. Be very afraid. You are probably in danger of repeating the torture you never resolved.

What was drawing me?
- On the surface, she was an attractive, upbeat, friendly person.
- She had similar interests—Coaching, nutrition, yoga, nature, writing, introspection, artsy stuff
- We had a very compatible sense of humor—we were often in peals of laughter over everything and nothing in particular
- She had some strengths I lacked that I could learn from—vegan cooking, physical therapy, little kids, working in hospice

What were the signs of trouble, where my radar alerts should have been going off [if I hadn't dulled them with over stimulation and craving factors]

- She was very seductive with friends—making me and everyone—male or female—feel like they were the "one" who made such a difference in her life, the one she could really open to, be herself with, share her deepest feelings—while she kept on her search discarding friendship suitors after a bite or two

- She started telling me about how this one and that one and the other one had dissed her, embarrassed her, asked too much of her, expected more than she or anyone in their right mind had to give.

- Now that should have stopped me in my tracks, don't you think? How was I NOT going to disappoint her, make her miserable and be the object of her life struggles?

- I was often the first to reach out. If I hadn't initiated communication, we probably would not have been in such frequent contact. Uhm, addiction alert? Are you noticing your behavior? Isn't it a little excessive?

- She was depressed a lot, even though she could appear bubbly and happy at moments when you first met her. My "this person needs to be rescued" alert should have been going off. Lots of people who communicate the need to be saved because they're drowning often elbow you in the face as you're trying to pull them out of deep water and back to shore.

- She did not follow through on her goals. In the short couple of years we were friends she backed out on half a dozen plans to be:
    - a yoga instructor
    - a physical therapist again
    - a Tai Massage Practitioner
    - a wellness coach
    - a weight loss coach
    - a Girl Scouts leader
- She was flirtatious with my husband. I tried not to notice, because that would have been much too uncomfortable for me. She had offered to do a Tai body massage with him after demonstrating how she did it on her own husband. I felt really embarrassed to be there when she was pushing on the inside of Jim's upper thigh, very close to his boys. There was no way I could not feel jealous or threatened with my friend touching MY guy like that. It was awkward and embarrassing enough being witness to how she touched her own man.
- She was very defensive and angry when called on anything by anyone. They were in the wrong. How could they misunderstand her so

badly? What idiots, bastards they were after all she had done for them!

- She coached for free and then resented it.
- She often disappeared even while we were in the same space, off in another world. Her eyes glazed over and she had to be pulled back with a louder voice, or repeated question.
- I attributed that to her being an "I" to my "E". I was just being a busy body "E" wanting to know what she was thinking, where she was going in her mind when she had a perfect right to privacy.
- That's all true in most cases; everyone has a right to their private thoughts. As long as they're not hidden thoughts that has to do with your relationship. She was holding her own uncomfortable feelings, not saying them, not giving us a chance to work them through until the pot bubbled over quenching the fire and it was too late to save the savory stew we thought we were cooking.

I'm sure there were MANY more cues that I chose to ignore, red flags that I pretended were surmountable. Watch out! Big bump ahead! Go very slowly or you'll have a blowout.

What's that queasy feeling you're having? Is it from you? Well yes of course it is, I'm having it. But where did it originate? What's wrong? This is a signal from yourself to take a step back and evaluate. Take some space, let things cool down. Did I do that? Clearly, if I did it was not enough.

# CHAPTER THIRTY-THREE

Lesson Five:
"Be your own best friend"

When I'm all alone with no one to play with, entertain me [well there is always Stewie]. I can always ask myself, what can we do today? I have lots of interests. Why not do that just "me and me"? Even going to a movie or taking myself out to lunch or taking myself for a ride.

In the last 6 months I've had the opportunity to get to know myself better. I feel proud of myself that I avoided trying to replace Jill with someone else. It's been a very long time, but I remember being the kind of girl who could not, NOT date. When I broke up with someone, I'd be on the prowl for a new boyfriend, going out with lots of people very quickly. I never gave myself much time to heal and evaluate what happened. That's very different in this case with Jill.

I retreated to myself as you have witnessed, crying, having mini tantrums, beating myself up, blaming her, BUT I didn't throw myself into finding another "best" friend. I used the opportunity to detox and refuel.

- Wrote about it
- Talked to my mentors about it
- Sunk into my husband's caring at critical moments
- Exercised
- Tightened up my nutrition
- Read lots of fun books to keep myself company
- Watched movies
- Took good care of my dogs
- Went for walks by myself
- Went to local meetings on different topics that I found interesting
- Concentrated my efforts on my work and coaching others
- Studied about Coaching, relationships, best practices, addictive friendships . . .

Then I began to ask myself what I would like to do, today—particularly on the rare days I had totally to myself. That might mean exploring some part of NH or Mass or Maine. It might mean taking me to dinner with my computer as a friend. That might mean . . . .

Creating an impromptu supervision group in the coaching academy on an interesting topic—like women's body images.

Or, starting a new course online to broaden myself?

Or asking Glenn to bring up the big easel from the basement to encourage myself to start painting again.

Or sitting outside and watching Stewie play in the yard.

Even though I'm usually a more social person, I found myself inviting myself to be with myself first.

During this time, I was invited to attend a spiritual medium training workshop as a receiver. I had been too nervous in the past to do anything like that, but the woman who invited me, Jenna, was so easy to be around, that I decided to take a risk. What could happen? What if a spirit did talk to me? Even though I'm pretty reluctant to believe that the dead talk to us through people, it was interesting and so I went.

* * *

"Tap, Tap, Tap . . . ." "Tap, Tap, Tap . . . ." The medium is telling us that while she is trying to pick up what the spirit "John" is communicating, she keeps hearing "Tap, tap, tap". The male "receiver's" eyes go round, as he tries to suppress the small smile that is spreading across his face. She describes his look and asks the receiver about different aspects of the man's home, his clothes, his interests and all the while "Tap, Tap, Tap . . . ." When she finishes with what she's gleaned from this visitation, she asks the receiver for feedback. He tells her she was "right on" in so much of what she told him, but most importantly, his father was a cobbler. Every time he repaired a heel, he would hammer it into the bottom of the shoe with a series of Tap, Tap, Tap's on each little nail.

I didn't realize it, but I had gone to this medium training workshop on my father's birthday.

There were 7 mediums and 7 receivers. Some readings were with the group of mediums focusing on the spirit of one receiver, as with the tapper. All of the mediums were trying to get messages from John, the father of the man in the room. One of them told him that he was to keep up the hard work. This meant something to the man whose eyes teared up. But he seemed most immersed and captivated when he heard about the "Tap, tap, tap". I have to say, that did give me a bit of a shiver. It was a very unusual thing to hear from a stranger.

After that pretty sensational demonstration, we started working in pairs. I was paired with Nicole an attractive tall young woman with long honey colored hair. We were supposed to say the name of a person we wanted to invite and no more. I decided on a man who had been in my life when I just graduated from college.

He was my boss and then my boyfriend for a short while. AND he was 27 years older than me.

She said, "I see someone, an older person . . . . He looks kind of grandfatherly. Does that make sense?" I was laughing inside, a bit embarrassed. "Yeah", I say. "That kind of makes sense." "He really cared about you, was very involved with you for a time," she continues. "And, uh . . ." she's almost blushing. She asks uncomfortably, "You had a special relationship with him?" "Well, yeah" I say, mirroring her discomfort. "That kind of relationship?" she asks softly, slowly. "Yeah, that kind of relationship", I stammer hoarsely, agreeing again but reflecting her discomfort and let out a little laugh to dispel some of it. "Ohhhh, well then that makes sense," she breathes deep into her abdomen.

"OK, he has something he wants to tell you. Annndd, I see a big green field . . . Why is he showing me this field? . . . He says, "It's ok, you no longer need to feel guilty."

This sends me into a reverie about the day we broke up. I lived with him for a very stabilizing year that got me back on my feet. Once I graduated, my parents decided to move back to South Jersey, leaving me alone in NY. I was pretty freaked out, not ready to live on my own yet, so I latched onto my boss who was very willing to take me on as his newest intern in work and love.

He was a very smart and funny and nice man. I learned a lot from him, but I wasn't in love with him. I felt very guilty about leaving because he was so attached to me.

I remembered the green field. It was in front of the house he had rented for us in the country. I told him I had to leave and dramatically ran out into the expanse of green, crying and tripping and falling into the grass, sobbing. I felt awful about hurting him, but had to leave before I was lost in his world with none of my own. We were both crying so hard that snot was running down both of our faces, seriously. I know that sounds disgusting and histrionic, but there it was. Seeing my upset, he pulled back his emotions, helped me up and let me leave. I knew I had broken his heart, but had to choose my own life over his. Always felt guilty about it.

Twenty years later, he called me to do a research project for him. It was a little awkward, but he was married to his 4th wife, who he claimed to adore and Glenn and I thought it was ok. It was a project on Catalina bathing suits; Focus Groups where women were shown a rack of suits as part of the project for their ideas. In focus groups, there are two rooms separated by a one way mirror, where those in the back can watch and listen to what's happening in the front room. Clients sit in the back, observing, taking notes, munching on M&M's, while the moderator—in this case me—runs the research session in the front.

At one point, I got a note from the backroom where he asked me to have them try on the suits. I was flabbergasted. He wanted to put up a screen in the room, have them go behind and change and come out to show us how the suits fit. OMG! Is he kidding!!!

These were not Sports Illustrated models who would be comfortable flaunting their bodies . . . well maybe one might have liked exhibiting herself, but the rest were normal figured flawed 30's-50's bodies like most of the rest of the world, who would have probably been mortified. More importantly, I was!

I began to remember that he WAS kind of lecherous and began feeling angry. I let him and the other men in the backroom know this was highly inappropriate and proceeded with the research as it was planned. I was judgmental and huffy and feeling like punishing him, justifying why it was for the best that I had left him so many years ago.

And, then the shocker, the bomb drop. As we were ending the project, wrapping up the report a couple of weeks later, one of the people in his office let it slip. He was dying. He had stomach cancer. There wasn't much time left. I wasn't supposed to know, but . . . he thought I might want to. I didn't know what to do, say, how to react . . . Really? Oh God, how awful. I realized, this was his way of seeing me one last time and saying goodbye, without trying to get me to feel sorry for him. New guilt on top of the guilt of hurting him so many years ago; Guilt for judging him; Guilt for realizing how important I must have been to him for him to create this bogus venue for saying goodbye with his dignity intact. I never said goodbye formally. Never acknowledged that I knew he was dying. I just sat with the sadness and guilt of being indignantly angry with him as part of our last encounters.

And, there I was in this room with Nicole telling me he said to drop the guilt.

Remember I said it happened to be my Dad's birthday? This man smelled like my Dad. I always think that we have our own tell-tale scents, but he smelled just like my Dad. Weird, right!? It actually got in the way of being close to him, because I was always aware of our age difference AND how he smelled like my Dad. So it was probably no coincidence that I thought about inviting him into the medium room on that day.

We all did some debriefing about our experiences, medium and receiver and then we switched. This time I was paired with Jenna. I know Jenna. She's the one who hosts the meetings. I have a feeling of trust with her even though I'm only a highly skeptical, partial believer in all of this. I had given Nicole a name and then might have been subtly communicating through my face and eyes information that could lead her one way or the other. Hot? Cold? Hot? Hotter?

So when I was paired with my friend, I got brave and still forgetting what day it was asked Jenna to invite my father into the space. Jenna is a medium AND a very entertaining channel who sings to you in an ethereal voice. She immediately started intoning, "Oh my darling daughter . . ." I was NOT even close to being my dad's darling, so I was very suspect, and kind of laughing to myself. But she kept chanting. Dad in Jenna's melodic voice told me how sorry he was for not being there for me. He kept apologizing in various versions while I drifted in my mind.

If he really was here, *he* SHOULD be apologizing. He was a very difficult father and person; Always moody and retreated or unpredictably explosive. I was terrified of him most of my younger life.

Uh oh . . . my peripheral vision is picking up a male presence. It's him, Tall, Dark and Smirking. Jenna's channeling is droning in the background as she sways in her seat, eyes closed. I whisper, in an annoyed voice, "What are you doing here, now?!"

He's wearing black jeans, black boots, a black biker T-shirt with a silver Harley on it and a condescending look on his face. He sounds like the Texan again.

"Ah came to protect you from all this nauseatin' goo."

"Nauseating?" "That my father wants to finally apologize?" I ask indignantly.

"Ya think that's yaw Dad?"

I, I stammer, "I don't know! But it's relieving to hear it anyway."

"Hhmmph" He snickers. "That's cheap."

"What?"

"That's all you need, is some spiritualist telling you Dad is sorry." He snorts. "Now, that's really rich."

"Well make up your mind. One minute cheap, the next rich!" I go into sarcasm as a defense.

"You think he's all sorry and healed because he's now in spirit? That's just too . . . ridiculous. Stories made up by you living types who are trying to get a life, but have no idea about reality." He snickers at me again.

"Stop. Why are you ruining this for me," I whine at him.

I realize that my face is flushed in annoyance and embarrassment at the same time. I never had the courage to consider my parents were actually reachable after they died and here I was taking a step towards allowing my feelings to be expressed when Magic Man appears to ruin it all.

What if it's just my imagination? What if this is all hokey and I'm using it as an avenue to letting something go. What's wrong with that?

As I was sitting in the mediums meeting, it occurred to me that my denial of death, that it won't happen to me was really the horrible thought that when I die I would have to see all the dead people who had tortured me in life—in particular my crazy grandmother, my mom and dad and a assorted other unpleasant types that I didn't want to associate with.

He drawls, "Well, relax. You're not going there. That's their destiny. Yours is much more interesting and you have a lot to do here before that anyway. WE have a lot to work on, right here."

"We?" I ask suspiciously, "Aren't you just a figment of my imagination?" And then I have a little giggle to myself. I can't use the word figment without wanting to say Fig Newton. I've always done that. I know, I digress to silliness at the most ludicrous moments.

He chuckles. "Yeah, it is a silly word."

"Stop reading my mind!"

"How can I read your mind, if I'm just a FIG Newton of your imagination?"

"You are soooo condescending", I sneer.

"Doesn't matter; I'm just here to keep you company on your journey and help to insure we get some things straight. And we can have some fun in the meantime."

I pretend not to pay attention and focus back on Jenna who is now saying that she has a message from Daddy for my sister. "He says to tell your sister that he's sorry for being hard on her too." I find myself bristling. Hard on her?! She was his little angel!!! But, of course, he couldn't or wouldn't let me think I was special to him, even for 2 minutes! He'd have to bring golden child back in!

"See what I mean? You need me. He's still trying to get his act together. But it's an act. Trust me. Don't bother. It's his journey. Yours is another, with me here right beside you." He's sitting on one of those fold up chairs that he brought out from a back room, long legs extended onto Jenna's lap. She doesn't notice.

"Would you take your legs off of her?" I hiss at him, trying no to interrupt Jenna's trance. "That's just disrespectful! And . . . wrong!"

He's behind me now with his hands warmly resting on my shoulders. "You're right. I'm sorry. We can talk later. Just don't get all soupy about your father. He's still the same guy that has nothing for you, dead or not."

Then I hear and see Jenna. She's smiling at me and talking, asking me a question that I can't quite make out, "Sharon, are you back?"

"Back?" I ask?

"Yes, you were murmuring something in what looked like a trance to me. Are you ok? Did your Dad say anything?"

I avoid the question. Instead, "I just realized, it's his birthday today."

"Ohhhh, no wonder his energy was so strong."

"Hhmmmpphhh."

I didn't know what to say. And I like her and want to be supportive of her entertainment factor. She's really adorable when she "channels".

She persists. "Did he say anything important? They usually want to tell you something when they come in that strongly".

"He said he was sorry. He called me his darling daughter." I mumble.

"Ohhhhhh. That's great. You know you've opened Pandora's Box. He's going to be coming in all the time now", she says with a self-satisfied smile on her face.

Ugh. I think to myself. What else will he want me to tell my sister?

I think I can hear "Tall, Dark, and Weird" snorting in the back of my mind.

Jenna is looking deep into my eyes. "What is it, she asks?"

Her eyes are soft melting pools of compassion. Whether I believe in mediumship or not I do believe in her. She's one of the most intuitive, alive, vibrant and caring people I've ever met.

Tears well up and leak out of the corners of my eyes.

"It's Dad . . . He was soooooo difficult and at times so scary. And he didn't like me." My eyes are now producing a steady stream of hot waterworks.

She reaches out and gently takes my hand.

That intensifies my pain, giving me permission to express it even though I know the people outside can probably hear me weeping. Her eyes soften and I think she's welling up too.

"He's sooooo sorry, Sharon. If he could do it over, he would. He said he's sorry he hurt you. That he was more taken with little Penchick . . ." I stop her.

"Wait, did you say Penchik?"

"Uhm . . ." She sits up straighter, eyes snapping open. "I'm not sure . . . Why?"

"You could not know that he called my sister that . . . That was a pet name he had for her."

She inhales deeply and smiles at me.

"And . . . ?"

"Maybe . . . he is . . . there . . . and sorry?" I feel like a five year old talking to my wise Aunt Jean.

Jenna squeezes my hand.

"Maybe he is." She smiles.

# CHAPTER THIRTY-FOUR

Lesson Six:
"Be the MOST gentle on yourself
when you make a mistake"

A long time ago my Mentor told me that the bigger the mistake, the gentler the intervention. I've learned how to do that with others much better than I've learned how to do that with myself. And, I have to admit, it's sometimes hard to remember to be nice when I feel self-righteously wronged.

But I do persist in being hard on myself as you can see from all I've shared with you. For someone who really can laugh at life's foibles I do take things very seriously and deeply.

Here's something you probably don't know about me, but maybe it will make sense from what you've learned about me so far. I am an immersion person.

When I'm learning something new, I tend to jump in and get totally involved. Well, that's what I did with Jill, right? I do the same with all things I find interesting and the more interesting the more I want to learn about it.

So it probably won't surprise you to hear that I went back to be a receiver again the following week. Jenna called me at the last minute and said she needed an extra receiver, might I be available and like to come. "Sure" I texted back. I was free for the evening, since Glenn needed to work on a book for the coaching academy.

I got there a few minutes ahead of time. Crystal was at the little table signing people in. She looked up at me with a smile, "You're almost ready, aren't you?" It was more of a statement than a question.

I looked back at her, eye brows raised in a question. "To be on this side . . ." she continued to smile.

I nodded, understanding. "How do you know?" I asked.

"It's your aura, it's swirling and active". Her eyes traced the perimeter of my shoulders and head.

"What are your gifts?" She asked in an encouraging voice.

"Gifts?" I asked myself if this was really relevant to me or was she projecting herself.

Wanting to feel included and in the spirit of the event, I surveyed myself. Hmmmm. "Well, I am pretty intuitive. You know, I'm pretty good at picking up on people's feelings. It's very useful in my work as a psychological interviewer."

"Do you visualize? How does it come to you?" She asks.

"Well, I am very visual in my imagination, but sometimes it's just having a sense or a thought." I explained.

"But you know, now that I'm thinking about it, I have on occasion picked up something and blurted it out without knowing why I said that particular thing. For example, a long long time ago, when I was a member in a therapy group, there was a woman who was soooooo annoying. I can't remember the specifics, but she was complaining and complaining and verbally attacking other people in the room, not being receptive to anything anyone in the room was saying, not even the therapist. It became difficult to listen to her, because there was no way of intervening, helping. She just got more and more ornery and offensive and left no room for anyone else to share their thoughts or issues. At one point, I had this overwhelming impulse and I shouted at her, 'Why don't you just jump out the window!'

Then I heard the words my mouth had just expelled and felt awful. I had never said anything like that to anyone before. I was kind of horrified with myself. She stared at me, with a look of shock and stammered,

'That's what my mother used to say.' It was kind of chilling and I really felt awful for saying it to her, but it stopped her in her tracks and she started talking deeply about the relationship with her mother. We were all able to breathe again."

"Yeah," Crystal nodded fervently. That's how it happens sometimes. Like a thought or expression from out of the blue comes into your mind."

"And, recently," I added. "I was doing an exchange with a massage therapist. She wanted help with her weight. We met at her office. When it was her turn on the table, I did a little Reiki with her and then took her on a guided meditation.

It was different than what I usually do. I usually just set up a passage way and have the client tell the story. But this time, I guided her to a field of wild blueberries, where she was picking them with a group of children from the school she worked in. They'd pick the berries and then take them to a waterfall to wash them before they ate them.

I finally let her take over the reverie. When we finished, she looked up at me and asked, 'how did you know about the blueberries? Did you see the painting I just did of the blueberry field? It's over there on the table.'

I didn't remember seeing a painting but thought to myself, "oh I must have picked it up subconsciously." I asked her where the painting was and she pointed to a table where I had put my purse. My purse was on top of a big piece of brown wrapping paper. I said, there's no painting here. She said, yes it's under that stack of papers. And it was, hidden from view.

It was a painting of a wild blueberry field that she used to play in when she was a child. If she got bored, her mother would send her out to pick berries. She loved the blueberry fields and she loved eating blueberries. I asked her if eating blueberries as a snack might help her with her weight loss goal.

Her eyes opened in excitement. "Yes! What a great idea!!" She was enthusiastic about it as a substitute for the sweets and starches that had crept into her life. And she actually did lose weight when I saw her a couple of months later."

"That's another great example. You are definitely displaying signs of psychic awareness. See you ARE almost ready." Crystal smiled at me with an acknowledging nod of her head.

I smiled back. There's a part of me that wishes psychic talents really did exist. I mostly believe in coincidence and people picking up on cues without realizing it. But the idea of a supernatural sense was romantic. So I said, "Well there were supposedly a number of gifted people in my family. My mother's older brother was able to read Kabala and foretold his death when he was only 15 years old. And my cousin could supposedly diagnose people medically through their energy."

Her eyes flared with the excitement of meeting a kindred soul. "You just have to open yourself and practice. Keep coming here and working with Jenna. It will help you open to your power." She beamed at me. I gave her my $20 for the medium event and took a seat.

After a short meditation introduction we were each paired with a medium for the first exercise. I got Anya, an enthusiastic but anxious woman with intense dark eyes. She was supposed to ask me who I wanted to talk to and then concentrate on me while doing spontaneous writing of what the spirit wanted to say to me.

I told her I wanted to talk to my mother. She stared at me for a minute, then closed her eyes, then stared at the paper in front of her.

"She was tall and thin?" She couldn't help herself. It was impossible for her to just write, she had to tell me what she thought she was hearing, seeing to get a read from me about whether or not she was going in the right direction.

I shook my head side to side. My mother was all of 4'9" and plump.

"She says you are very loved." Ok, Nice to know.

"She says to tell you she's still in the chair." Really, what chair? Then I think about my grandmother who was always in the recliner chair staring at the TV set, jaw dropped as she snored, with her upper false teeth falling down to meet the lowers. Not the prettiest sight. Was it Grandma coming through? Weird if so . . . . And, she was not a very pleasant person! I wasn't sure I wanted to contact her. In my mind I thought, Grandma, get out of the way. Let Mom come through. If you have something to say, you can tell me another time, ok?!

The medium kept reaching for images or messages, but none of them made sense. My mind started wandering. I started seeing slowly swirling mists wrapping loosely around her arms. They continued up to her shoulders and then converged behind her in the form of a graceful ethereal mist woman with long white hair and billowy long skirt as if she was standing in a wind. I couldn't make out the details. Everything was filmy whites, pale grey and blue. I couldn't see her face, just a kind of benign presence and smile with soft eyes.

I said to the medium, interrupting her guesses, "I see a beautiful woman in a diaphanous dress standing behind you. She's got a soft smile on her face and she's kind of illuminated but I can't make out her exact features. It's kind of foggy or filmy."

"Really?" she asked, stopping her focus on trying to find my Mom. Her voice lilted. "That's my guide! I can't believe you can see her!! Did she say anything? She never says anything to me, just looks at me with those

SHARON LIVINGSTON, Ph. D.

sweet soft eyes. I keep hoping she's going to tell me something."

"Have you asked her anything?"

"Well, no. I didn't want to impose my will, hoping she'll just tell me what she thinks I need to know . . ."

I look at the shimmery image behind her who is nodding at me with an encouraging smile.

"I think she wants to know what you want to know from her."

"Really!?! Ohhh . . . Well, I want to know, am I on the right path to be a great medium?"

I look back to the ghostly figure. She continues to shimmer but there is no change, no expression, just a kindly presence.

"Ask her something else . . ." I suggest.

"Ohhh", She takes a deep breath. "Will my psychic ability become an important part of my career?"

My eyes return to the beautiful specter. I can't believe but I can actually see her roll her eyes while maintaining a smile on her pale glistening lips.

"Not clear", I tell her.

"Uhmmm, do you think I should lose a little weight?" I stifle a laugh. Clearly Anya could lose 30-40 lbs.

The lovely vision suddenly erupts with vibrant color—lavish purples and pinks and blues in her gown, golden hair, and intense aqua eyes, rich ruby lips forming the word YES that billows out in a giant word bubble and bursts over Anya's head.

Anya looks surprised. "OMG, she does think I'm fat!!" Her eyes look like they are tearing up.

"Are you OK?" I ask, concerned

"Yes," she replies with a combination of annoyance, rebelliousness and a sense of resolution.

"Honestly, I think she's been trying to tell me that for a long time but I haven't been listening. I keep thinking there's something more intriguing, more spiritual that she would have to share with me. But I guess I have to deal with my worldly body."

"Well, you know what they say, first things first," I say in what I hope sounds like a sweet tone trying to lighten up the moment. "Maybe we need to have our earth bodies in alignment before we can get the answers to the more otherworldly questions?"

"Yes. That makes sense. I hate the way I look. I guess I thought guides and spirits would see my essence and not my physical self".

"Maybe they'll be better able to see your essence when it's unencumbered with negative self-concepts from your view of yourself," I try to help.

"Yeah, I've always hated the way I look. The kids always made fun of me. And now, here I am as an adult, still making fun of myself. You should hear what I say to myself in the mirror in the morning when I'm brushing my teeth. I actually try not to see myself, because I don't want to see how fat I am."

"Oh, Anya, I'm so sorry. You seem like a lovely person. Look at those bright sparkly eyes of yours. You could look at how pretty they are when you brush your teeth and say nice things to yourself every morning."

"I know . . ." she says sadly.

"You know what? I just so happen to help people with eating issues. Would you like to consider letting me help you?"

"OMG, I hear her saying, "Yes!" She says, somewhat surprised.

I look up and see a bunch of "Yes" balloons bursting over Anya's head and a clear huge glistening red grin on the spirit's otherwise transparent face.

"I can give you my card, and you can contact me. My office is just a couple of miles from here . . . ."

"Will she help me find my psychic capabilities if I lose the weight?" She asks hesitantly.

I start to say I don't know about these things, when I feel a tap on my left shoulder and the slightest breezy whisper in my ear, "tell her yes I will."

I look at the would-be-medium and say confidently, "I believe she will, Anya."

Anya looks relieved and then a little excited. She says, "OK, I'm going to do it. Please may I have your card? I know she sent you to me and I'm going to lose this weight and negative self-concept once and for all!"

"OK," I say, reaching into my purse and searching for a card. "OK, I'd be happy to help you."

# CHAPTER THIRTY-FIVE

Lesson Seven:
"Life is an adventure"

There's always something new to learn. There's always a new story. And, good stories have a beginning, middle, a problem, and a satisfying resolution. Expecting to go through life without problems is a recipe for depression.

The problems actually make it more exciting. You can't enjoy sweet without a little sour or salty or bitter. It's about balance. But the aspect that is temporarily out of balance, the problem, makes it exciting. Makes you want to get back into balance. Makes you become a detective searching for a solution, the missing piece to the puzzle.

I lay in my bed at the end of a long day. It felt so good to feel the soft cool sheets as I slid my legs under the velvety comforter and lowered my head into the fluff of the down pillows. I took a deep breath and let out a long sigh. I love getting into bed after a long hard day and feeling the luxury of sinking into relaxation. Glenn was getting settled on his side. He turned off the light, snuggled his back into my left side and we wished each other sweet dreams.

Sweet dreams, I mused as I absently scratched his back. Gosh I hadn't had ANY dreams in weeks. What was up with that?! I have always felt good about the fact that I dream frequently and find my dreams to be creative at worst, and full of interesting codes and ideas at best.

Creative at worst—HUH! I've had some terrifying dreams that were very imaginative but also unpleasant. Still, not dreaming was disappointing. I enjoy the puzzle of my dreams. I often write them down and do some form of dream work on them. There are a number of different techniques. I like doing a Gestalt analysis of dreams, where each element of the dream represents an aspect of self. You start by saying the dream in the first person. That in itself is often revealing of part of the message of the dream. You then "become" each part of the dream and describe it. E.g., I am the house. I am large with many rooms. I have many things hidden in me, all of them interesting although sometimes hard to find. I'm sturdy and protective . . .

You get the idea. You can then have various elements talk to each other. For example, the house and plush sofa converse:

House—Hi

Sofa—Hi. Thanks for keeping me safe and dry and soft.

House—Why, you're very welcome. I much prefer to have a soft and supple sofa inside me, so I'm delighted that I can keep you dry.

Sofa—And I'm glad you keep out intruders. I'm very fussy about who I allow to enjoy me.

House—As it should be. I do work hard to ensure only those welcome, come inside.

Etc.

This was not part of a dream I had, but it's interesting that even as I made this up, I realized that the sofa was a feminine part of me. I was seeing the color purple. The house was an older protective male— sturdy, solid, well built, impervious to all but the most deliberately aggressive attempts to enter.

When the two parts talk, the conversation continues until it comes to an end that makes sense in some way. The results can be surprising, entertaining, scary, but always very revealing. I find it very helpful in understanding something about myself or a client and useful in identifying solutions. There are actually accounts of famous inventions and solutions that resulted from dreams:

- The tune for "Yesterday" came to Paul McCartney in a dream
- How Google was born—The April 9, 2012, edition of Fortune magazine shared a story of how Larry Page one of the founders of Google dreamed of "downloading the entire web onto computers" when he was 23 years-old. He said, "I spent the middle of that night scribbling out the details and convincing myself it would work."
- The story of Frankenstein came to author Mary Shelley in a dream
- Elias Howe came up with the sewing machine while dreaming
- Einstein dreamed his theory of relativity—$E=MC^2$
- DNA was discovered in a dream
- And, there are many, many more instances of problem solving while sleeping

So because I think dreams are so powerful and important, that night when I fell asleep I invited myself to remember a dream. I woke up at 3 am, looked at the clock, scanned my thoughts and realized I couldn't remember any dreams. Disappointed I got up to use the bathroom. Might as well! Maybe I'll sleep a little longer, if Stewie doesn't wake me up to take him out. Got back into bed and quickly fell back to sleep . . . .

*I am standing outside in the driveway next to the fence that separates the asphalt from the backyard. I am waiting for Stewie to find his spot. He's doing his typical sniff, sniff here, sniff, and sniff there. I'm waiting for him to do that silly thing he does just before he's ready to squat. He starts running at full speed to a sudden stop where he assumes the position. Weird what you get to know about critters you spend a lot of time with. A car drives up behind me and stops. I turn to see Jill standing there. She looks at me with a sad, slightly shy but warm expression, head down a little, peering at me from beneath her slightly raised eyebrows, perhaps to see how I respond. I am surprised to see her; happy to see her, scared to see her. She says, "I really miss you," with an imploring tone. "I miss you, too," I answer tentatively, nervously with a mixture of sadness, hope and cautiousness.*

*She comes closer and we both peer into an old dumpster that is standing here. I didn't notice it before, but here it is. I realize it has been here for quite a while. Strange, but the waste management people have not emptied it out completely. There are things on the bottom from a long time ago. I see my red faux alligator purse that I haven't used since Jill and I stopped talking. It's lying on top of a discarded corrugated box. And a foot away, growing mold in the wet smelly residue is an orangey brown purse, very similar to my red one; it used to be Jill's. I look up at her to see her reaction . . . . And I wake up.*

Wow. I finally had a dream. And how interesting! Our purses!? Mine thrown away but retrievable! Hers immersed in the putrid muck. Ha! My aggressive part has a sense of humor!! Obviously still mad at her, I made the thing that represented her, gross and stinky. Something about my premature toilet training must be evident in my dreamwork sarcasm. Can't help but laugh at myself even though the memory of her face tugs at my heart.

So in Gestalt Dreamwork, after telling the dream, you identify with each part as if it's yourself. Ugh. I have to be the gross brown purse too?! Yech.

But let's try . . .

Red faux alligator purse: "I am easy to take with you because I'm compact, but I carry lots of things, money, credit cards, lipstick, receipts, and notes. I'm a pretty color. I'm good quality but not costly. I look more expensive than I am, so I put on a good show even though I'm not really alligator. If I were alligator, I'd be dangerous. But I'm not. I just look tough. Really, I'm easy to get along with and I am durable. I've been around a long time. Can't understand why I've been discarded when I'm in perfectly good shape. I'm not sure what's inside me. Maybe a few coins, or a couple of dollars, but no credit cards. Maybe some old charge slips or notes. My clasp works well. I hope Sharon fishes me out and starts using me again."

Orangey brown purse: "Uch, I'm all dirty and gross. What am I doing in here? This is disgusting. I'm an unattractive color. I know someone must like my color or I wouldn't have been created like this, but I hate sitting in this mildew and mold water. It's going to make me rot. No one will want me. I'll really get discarded into some junk pile or garbage dump. There's nothing inside me. I'm empty and useless. I wish I didn't know what I was."

Dumpster: "I'm a big dark grey dumpster. I'm brought in when people have a lot to throw away. I'm very strong and easy going. I can take whatever you've got and I don't have any feelings about it one way or another. Bring it on. I'll just sit here until they take me away and then send me elsewhere. It doesn't matter to me. I'm hard to move though. It takes a big truck and heavy duty lift to cart me away. I'll stay with you as long as you want, take whatever you have to get rid of. When I'm full, I'll get emptied out and start all over again. Don't feel bad if I can't take anymore at a given moment. As soon as I'm emptied I'll be back if you need me."

Residue at the bottom of the dumpster: "I'm a bunch of waste sitting here; I'm made up of rain water, mold, box parts and some other malodorous stuff. And oh yeah, there are a couple of purses here too. I smell like the contents of a dumpster that's been behind a restaurant in NYC in the summer time. I'm not supposed to be here. I was supposed to have moved on many months ago, but here I sit. It's uncomfortable to be me because I know I'm not appealing and no one wants me around. I make them look bad. I used to be useful, but not anymore."

Garbage Man Who Left the Residue: "Hey, I'm just doing my work. I pick the thing up and dump it out as best I can. Don't check the bottom. If something's stuck, it's stuck. What do I care? I get paid for moving these big muthas and turning them over. That's it. I don't look. I don't care. It's enough that I have to get my hands dirty and smell all this stuff. I don't complain, so don't come crying to me."

Asphalt: "Is this a joke. Ass Fault. It's not my fault. I'm just the driveway. I allow people to come and go to this house. I take a lot of beating from cars and trucks and those rotten mutts go all over me. And do I complain? Nooo. I don't ask for anything. You'll just use me up until I need to be replaced. I get it."

Stewie: "I'm an adorable dog. I'm a cute Shih Tzu. Everyone thinks I'm precious. I look like a girl to some people but I'm really a tough little guy. The only one who's really allowed around me is my mom. I tolerate everyone else, but don't be fooled. It's me and Mom to the end. I love running around the backyard. There's so much to explore and sniff and pee on. This is serious business you know. I can tell who and what has been here through my incredible sense of smell. It's important to leave my mark to let people know that I own this place and my Mom, of course."

Sharon: "I'm standing here watching Stew and his machinations. He's so funny in his marking and bio habits. It looks like it's fun to him. I'm glad it's not too hot, but I wish it was autumn already. I'm standing here in my little striped Express dress, barefoot on the driveway. I'm a little bored. Wish I had something fun to do. Just have to enjoy the moment . . . and Stewie".

Jill: I'm not sure why I'm here. I guess it's hard to believe that Sharon hasn't responded to my sweet note to her. I had to see what was up. I feel tentative about being here, but I want to know she still loves me even if I have nothing to give her back. She just expects too much, and I don't have that much to give to her. I don't know why. But why do I have to? It just is. I'm at peace with it and have to move on. But then why am I here? Did I come on my own accord? Maybe she summoned me. Yes that's it. She made me come. She threw out her psychic magnet and drew me in. I'll leave in a moment. I don't want that old purse anymore, anyway. I actually forgot about it."

Back to dreamwork process. Have the elements talk to each other.

RED Purse: "Wow, what happened to you. You look and smell pretty bad."

Orangey Brown Purse: "Oh shut up. You were just lucky to be perched on that box. I wish someone had knocked YOU into the muck and left me high and dry."

RED Purse: "Sour grapes."

Orangey Brown Purse: "You better believe I'm sour. I can hardly stand myself".

RED Purse: "Well at least you have a sense of humor."

Orangey Brown Purse: "Don't count on it. I'm pretty disgusted with everything."

RED Purse: "Well if they fish me out of this prison, I'll try to get them to rescue you too."

Orangey Brown Purse: "Yeah, why?"

RED Purse: "Because, you may be perfectly fine once you get washed up and someone could put you to good use."

Orangey Brown Purse: "Grumble, grumble"

RED Purse: "what's that you say?"

Orangey Brown Purse: "You look so pretty and I'm a mess."

RED Purse: "You're right, I was just lucky. I could have been just like you, it was just the luck of the draw."

Orangey Brown Purse: "Well thanks for saying that. I would appreciate if you could get me out of here too. I do like being useful."

RED Purse: "I'll do my best. I promise."

Sharon: "Hey."

Jill: "Hi."

Sharon: "Why are you here?"

Jill: "Honestly, I'm not sure. And it's your dream, so maybe you know better than I do."

Sharon: "Maybe I want to tell you something or hope you wanted to tell me something."

Jill: "I told you. I'll always love you and Glenn and Stewie and Zach, but it just doesn't work. I don't know why. And it doesn't matter why. Let's just move on".

Sharon: "Then why do you keep coming back? I don't believe it's just me sucking you in!"

Jill: "Because it WAS fun for awhile. I really did enjoy talking with you and laughing with you. But . . . ."

Sharon: "But what?"

Jill: "I'm probably just not a good friend for you. You want too much. You want me to understand my discomfort with real friendship and I just can't. I want lots of friends who don't make demands on me. I can be very close and intimate in the moment, but then I need space. I'm an "I." I need my I time. I don't want you to be so important to me. I don't want anyone to be that important to me. I do the right thing, saying my kids and husband are that important, but not really. No one is. I can't allow that. It's too risky, too scary, I couldn't bear being the one rejected."

Sharon: "It does suck."

Jill: "I'm sorry. I never meant to hurt you."

Sharon: "I believe that."

Jill: Silence

Sharon: "Do you wanna know what the worst part is?"

Jill: "ok."

Sharon: "The worst part is that I can't fix it. I've always had the belief that if I make a mistake there's something I can do to repair it. It's sooooo hard for me to believe that wanting you and worrying about you was such an impossible error that you would not want to try to work it out to remain friends.

I know I have the capacity to change my behavior. If you said, 'Hey, let's cut back on the texting, or let's have a plan to meet once every couple of weeks', that would have been workable . . . . I dunno.

Maybe I'm kidding myself. I wanted you as a best friend who I could communicate with several times a week or more. That wasn't what you wanted.

The truth is I can't change who I am. I'm great in a lot of ways as a friend, but I do expect something in return. I really wanted you to be my best friend, my real friend. When you said I could call on you anytime I thought you meant it. The one time I did, it was the wrong time. I understand. You were trying hard to be grown up while you were alone for 10 days. Instead of encouraging you in a way that felt good to you, I needed help and worried when I didn't hear from you. You wanted to know that you could confidently leave and have fun with your kids without anyone doubting you.

SHARON LIVINGSTON, Ph. D.

I don't attach to people that easily. I love lots of people. I have lots of people I'm friendly with, but I really thought we were true friends, to the moon and back, to infinity. Once in a blue moon I feel the connection that I felt with you. Call it chemistry or unconscious reaching out to unconscious. We recognized something in each other that drew us together. You were much more like my family. And I guess there was the problem. I was repeating the faulty relationship in my family. I guess we all repeat the problem until we finally work it through. It still hurts to think we can't.

You were and probably always will be special to me. I wish I could fix my part. But that doesn't mean I have magic or can control yours. It's still sad so many months later."

Pregnant pause . . . .

Jill: "Can I go now?"

Ugh. Even in a dream, I've held her captive, against her wishes. Sometimes, it's very hard to be me.

I looked up the meaning of "purse" in a symbolic dream dictionary.

### Purse

*If you lost a purse in your dream, this signifies disappointment with a friend or lover.*

*To see or carry a purse in your dream represents secrets, desires and thoughts which are being closely held and guarded. It symbolizes your identity and sense of self. Consider also the condition of the purse for indications of your state of mind and feelings.*

*To dream that you lost your purse denotes loss of power and control. You may have lost touch with your real identity. To dream that you lost your purse, but find the contents of what is inside means that what matters and what is important is what's inside. You need to look past the exterior and focus on the inside. To see an empty purse represents feelings of insecurity or vulnerability.*

What **IS** my real identity . . . !?!

# CHAPTER THIRTY-SIX
## "Do You Have A BFF → BFN Story?"

Hey. How's it going? I realized that I'm always telling you about me and my travails, but never ask you about you. And, you know, I don't even know who you are or why you picked up this book and decided to read it, read me. And, I am interested. If you've gotten this far, there's something compelling about my story that's kept you reading. I'd love to know about it.

What did it make you think? Feel?

How do you relate to what I've been going through?

What's **YOUR** story? You can email me or call me and tell me about it.

Maybe you'll be part of my next book! Anonymous of course! But maybe it will be a detox for you, too. I know I've changed and healed in this flow of thoughts and feelings and disappointments and observations.

If you're up to it, interested, you can email me DrSharonLivingston@gmail.com. Or call (603) 537-0775 and leave a voice message.

So would you like to hear my latest?

I've decided to work with a trainer. I'm great at doing cardio, but my upper body is a wimp. It's amazing that I can bring the heavy bags of groceries up from the garage. Well not that bad, but my arms and shoulders and back are definitely not in league with my legs. My legs are powerful, they are strong and streamlined, ready to go on a second's notice. They can sprint or steadily take me for miles. My arms on the other hand [Ha! Pun! So silly you are, Sharon!], are weak and flabby, making me want to hide them under sleeves. It's as if my arms and legs belong to different people.

So it was time to bring my parts together. My Chiropractor suggested Rhodiola, no, not the herb that provides energy, but a woman around the corner from his office who he said was an extraordinary trainer. Her mother must have been a hippy to name her after a plant, but, hey, if she can rev me up I don't care what her name is. Not sure what they call her for short, Rhodi, Rhod, Ola, Olay. I've been calling her Rho; Reminds me of a rowing machine which is great for my upper body and torso; Works for me.

I've had four sessions with her so far. Each time she gets me to work some other set of muscle fibers that I'm acquainted with and those who it seems I've never met before. Introductions can be awkward; sometimes you don't know how to behave with a stranger, right? Well, one set of dwarfed triceps strands in my left arm got particularly upset with me for pushing them beyond their comfort zone. I don't know about you, but the second day after a set of new exercises is my biggest pain point and then it settles down.

On Monday, Rho had me do something different with upper body and arms. Honestly, I can't even remember specifically what it was. Tuesday I had normal soreness, even Wednesday when it should have peaked, my left arm was achy but not out of the ordinary for a second day recovery. Then Thursday came. OMG! The pain!!!!

The oddest thing is to realize what muscles we use without paying much attention. We do it automatically. And, even more interesting is to notice the actions we do with those muscles that we may not have realized. When my left triceps close to my elbow was so unhappy and full of lactic acid I couldn't fully lift turn and bend my arm without intense pain—I mean so intense that I actually yelped a few times, I couldn't help but turn my awareness to what it was trying to do. Perhaps, more disconcerting than the instant agony in my arm was the realization that I frequently flipped my hair.

Really?! The Hair-Flip! Me? Now, you have to understand that I have never in the past and still do not consider myself to be a girly girl. When I first got into therapy, I described myself as a little boy who grew into a woman. Not even a Tomboy, just a shy, nerdy little boy. Then I was an overweight teenager, trying to become invisible in a cloak of fat. So I never developed a particularly feminine self-concept even though I kind of know I'm an attractive woman, now. But I do know that when I see girls/women do the hair flip I silently chuckle to myself because it's such a female power move. It can mean several things. For example:

- A hair flip in the presence of a guy is an indication of sexual interest—like an entranced person baring her neck to a seducer in True Blood or some other Vampire fantasy. This type of hair flip may be accompanied by a shy or sexy gaze back to the other from beneath lowered lids and slightly bent head.

- A hair flip can be a show of feminine superiority to other women—I'm sexy and therefore powerful and you're not. This flip is seen along with a proud and arrogant rising of a jutted out chin.

- A hair flip can also be a sign of dismissal—shrugging off or discarding an unwanted overture or thought, feeling or belief that goes along with looking away.

On Thursday, I must have reached up to do the hair flip at least 20 times. Each time I tried I was punished with a radiating wrench of pain that almost took my breath away. Twenty times!? Maybe more!? Really, I flip my hair all day long and don't even know it? This was more shocking than the spasm of pain.

I looked up "Hair Flip" in the Urban Dictionary on the internet.

> "*The act of flipping hair to move on from a failed relationship*", is suggested and depicted by Chris Crocker (several times) in his YouTube video The Hairflip.
> *Chick:* "I hate my ex, Chris, what do I do?!"
> *Chris:* "If ya best friend stole ya man, say you know what? She can have my man but she can't have my hair extensions, and you flip that hair until that bitch is gone, outta ya mind. It ain't no thang, it's a hairflip!"

What am I flipping off? Am I still metaphorically giving Jill the hair flip? Am I doing it so frequently because it's so hard to let go, that I have to reject my impulses over and over? Is this just repeating the pain or finally working it though?

The pain in upper arm was so bad that I went to see Doc Dillon the chiro. Actually, I asked him about my arm when I took Stewie for his doggie L4 adjustment.

He assured me it was just a muscle. Today, Saturday, I can flip my hair with ease. Yay!!!! I wonder how many times I'll flip something off today. I know I won't know because with my triceps healed, my attention will go elsewhere. Do I have some other girly girl affectations, behaviors that I'm not aware of? Even though I may have had disparaging thoughts of feminine women who I thought leveraged their wiles, I'm kind of intrigued. What if I allowed myself to think of myself as truly feminine? What might that mean?

One meaning of "purse" in the symbolic dream dictionary is vagina. The pretty purse I discarded but was still intact might be part of my feminine identity? Without a strong identification with a mother figure, is it hard to feel ones feminine muscle? Jill so much represented my magical mommy; losing her felt like losing my mother, again. Finding myself alone but unscathed in the dumpster may be a way of reclaiming myself?

Sharon, I give you permission to be the beautiful, functional life container that you are, to claim your identity.

# CHAPTER THIRTY-SEVEN

What a crazy week. A couple of months ago, I had enrolled in and paid for a *Train The Trainer* program so I could teach hypnosis, not just perform it as I have been doing for four years. It would be a great addition to the work we were doing at the academy. So many people were interested in learning and had been asking about it.

NGH—The National Guild of Hypnotists—offers these intensive, 5 day programs once a year in Marlboro MA, just an hour from where I live in NH. The timing was perfectly nestled between a research project on skin care and a set of new coach the coach sessions I had scheduled. NGH has figured out over the years that they get the best participation by starting on Sunday and going till Thursday as a pre-convention offering. The three day yearly convention starts on Friday. It's an 8 day immersion in all forms of hypnosis, NLP, meditation, healing with scientists, doctors and creative artists and metaphysical types converging to learn and share and party. I'm not really the party type, so I go home in the evenings.

I was very much looking forward to the entrancement of a class. Such fun to learn more! Then two weeks before, the schedule of my skin care project changed. One day was now going to take place on the Monday of my class, but in Chicago. I almost cried when I got the news of the time and place change. I couldn't tell my client, "No." [I have trouble saying no, in general, but this is a big client who I didn't want to disappoint AND research projects pay a lot more than coaching does.] At first, I didn't know what I was going to do. There was no refund, and the course was $2,000. After wringing my hands, I decided to call the instructor and just put it out on the table, "Could I make up a day somehow if I missed the Monday and came a little late on Tuesday?" We talked about it and he said, "Yes". Phew!!! What a relief!

But, as I said earlier, what a crazy week! I left my house at 6:30 am on Sunday morning to get to the class, packed bags, computer, low fat, low carb protein snacks in tow. When I go to these kinds of events, I have to bring my own food options, because they are overwhelmingly under supplied with healthy things to eat or snack on. And I have to chew new thoughts over in a new learning environment. If I don't have my own stash, I end up eating whatever is there and come back 5 lbs. fatter and miserable. So I was toting a lot along with me, which made for a more intense planning and packing experience. It also makes me more anxious.

On Saturday, I went for a massage and actually had an anxiety attack on the table. That's just wrong, isn't it? You go for a massage to relax the kinks out of your body and mind, right? At least I do. I was laying there, doing a little self-hypnosis, letting myself sink into the table beneath me, feeling body getting heavier and heavier, when all of a sudden a wave of fear gripped me, starting in my abdomen and traveling up to my chest and throat. I tried to stay calm and ignore it, breath into it, but the adrenalin had taken over and my legs began to shake. Elaine, my massage therapist couldn't help but notice. She questioned me about it—You OK? Your face is red and your legs are trembling."

Ugh. So embarrassing . . . . I've had anxiety and panic attacks since I was five, going back to my Aunt Jean's house with her and her husband to spend a week with them. We were in the Lincoln Tunnel traveling from South Jersey to their apartment in Brooklyn. We came to a standstill in traffic behind an accident. We were stuck there for an hour. I was fine at first then started feeling confined and aware of the fumes and that we were under water. I began to feel claustrophobic and then terror overtook me. I feel sorry for my aunt. She had no idea of what to do with me as I screamed and sobbed until we were finally able to move and see the light at the other side.

Elaine remained calm. She said, "You're probably dehydrated. Here, sit up for a moment and have some water." I shakily, but dutifully obeyed. I lay back down and she continued with the massage, speaking to me soothingly about nothing in particular, which did seem to calm me down. A little while later, a second wave struck. I asked her for more water, sat up, sipped, took a deep breath, and we were able to finish the session.

I got through the rest of the day, telling myself I was probably anxious about the combined trip. Honestly, as much as I LOVE my work, I HATE traveling. What used to be a nice experience changed dramatically after 9-11. I hate the long lines, the metal detectors, the scanners and "I'm only going to touch your private parts with the back of my hand." And of course, I often get called out for the scan. So demeaning to be felt up in public . . . .

Anyway, I kept my nervousness to myself so I wouldn't upset my hubby, who also hates when I leave, and prepared and packed so I could just slip out of the house on Sunday morning.

I had one wave of fear soon after I sat down in the class. It was another intense wave from abdomen up, my head felt hot, again shaking and weak kneed. I texted my naturopath under the table and briefly told him what was happening, asking if we could talk. Ugh, interrupting him on a Sunday morning?! He texted back, "Can't talk; in church. I'll call you when I get out." I kept breathing and took notes to put my mind on something else while in the back of my mind I worried about the worst. Am I having a stroke? Do I have a brain tumor? It's never something manageable like I caught a little bug or I'm having an allergic reaction. I always skip to the end.

Finally the phone vibrated and lit up. I tried to sneak out of the room as quietly as possible. There was a stairwell just outside so I opened the heavy solid steel door and took the call there hoping it would serve as a sound barrier. I recounted my symptoms and he said, "It's just your thyroid. Stop taking your thyroid supplement. When did you take it last?"

"This morning around 6, just before I left for Marlboro."

"It will take a while to get out of your system, but you'll feel much better later and tomorrow. I'm seeing you next week, right?"

"Yes on Tuesday."

"Let me know how you feel later and tomorrow. Probably reduce your dose or just don't take it until we see how much you need. AND jot down every supplement you're taking and send to me."

He knew that I was a supplement junky who sometimes added my own concoctions to what he prescribed. Well . . . not prescribed exactly, vitamins are over the counter, but recommended.

"It may be that you're taking something that's over activating the thyroid."

"You know, I've been taking that Isagenix Cleanse for Life product that I showed you. That's been kind of new."

"That could do it. It has pretty impressive ingredients that may have adjusted your thyroid function so you need less."

"That's very cool" I said feeling a little excited that maybe this was actually a sign of something improving. "So I can go to Chicago? I'm sooooo shaky."

"Yes, you'll be fine. Make sure to keep your protein up. The extra thyroid seems to be pushing you into hypoglycemia. So eat protein and veggies and a little fruit in small quantities throughout the day. Ok?"

I calmed down and agreed, said good-bye and reached for the door. It was locked. Ugh. I had to walk down a flight to an exit that put me on a dirt path to an open field that looked nothing like the setting of the hotel. It took me awhile to reorient myself and then I realized I was in the back of the building, having to walk through dirt and then wet grass. Great for my high heeled sandals, yuch!

"H-e-y", I heard a drawl and looked around to see my Texan magic man leaning up against the outside stucco wall chewing on a long blade of grass.

"Hey", I answered. "Is that western dental floss or something?"

He tipped his hat, "You are the sarcastic kind, ain't you Ma'am?"

"What are you doing here?"

"I think the more important question is what y'all are doing here?" he drawled.

I fussed at him. "How about having an anxiety attack, too much thyroid, scared of being outside my normal environment for a week and then locked out of this workshop! I can't believe the door locked and I couldn't get back in! How'd ya make that happen?"

"I heard you callin' for me . . . "

"Are you nuts?" I indignantly responded. "You're the last thing I need now. If anyone sees me talking to you they'll think I'm crazy!"

"Nah just entranced."

"So why might you want to talk to me?" He goaded me, "Isn't that one of those questions you train your people to ask, when they won't answer?"

"Ugh! You are impossible. I mean you really are impossible and I'm delusional.

OK, let me go with this . . . You're some kind of waking dream reflection of something . . . . So I might as well take the opportunity to look deeper . . . .

I got scared, felt lonely and isolated, and feel wimpy and childlike, so I brought in a hero to save me."

"Uh huh . . ." he nodded slowly encouraging me to continue.

"Maybe I saw this wet grass and wanted to be rescued. If I could conjure up someone like you, maybe I could magically transport myself back to the front of the hotel without ruining my shoes or twisting an ankle . . ."

"Now how would that look, you suddenly appear in front of the hotel. You'd freak people out. Can't have that; you'd be even more scared outa yaw wits, trying to explain the unexplainable."

"Maybe I just missed you . . . You know, wondering if you were ever going to come back. Wanting to know more about who, what you are, and what you represent if you're just a reverie."

"I'm a fig newton of your imagination, huh?" he snickered.

"I should never have told you that", I flushed in embarrassment and annoyance.

"Probly not." He drawls.

"I needed some reinforcement to get me through this class while I'm feeling so vulnerable. I'm so tired of having to leave home to work. I really need to convince my research clients to do the work remotely. It's sooooo much better for everyone. No one has to travel and we wouldn't have to pay people as much. Would save the companies so much time and money . . . . Reports would get done faster. We could interview people in their own environments which could yield more realistic results . . ."

"Y'all don't have to convince me. I personally would just beam us right there, if you were up to it. But that's another story."

"Oh right. I can see my landing page, now. Star Trek Research—brings a whole new meaning to a beaming interviewer. Why is this woman beaming? Because she can bring you results straight from the source, getting reality based results, faster, more efficiently with less cost to you in people power and travel bills."

"Wellll, if you ask me, and I know you didn't, that's pretty lame. But we could work on that if you really wanted to. I know how to transmute within the flexible boundaries of the space time continuum. It's science. You know, magic is science before its time and all that."

"Tssscccch!" I had no words, just eye rolling annoyance as I headed into the wet grass. I looked over my shoulder to see if he was coming, but he was nowhere to be seen.

I heard a whisper in my ear like the wind through trees. "See, you miss me already."

I hrrrrmmmphed and kept stepping my way through the sod.

Took ten minutes to get around the hotel and back to my workshop. I was embarrassed to have interrupted the class and sheepishly took my seat.

The rest of the day went well. It was all very interesting, being reminded about the value of hypnosis, how to test for receptivity of the subject, which kind of inductions to use, how to create focus and attention, and how attending to something takes you away from worry. That was just what I personally needed. I attended to the class and my anxiety subsided.

Later that afternoon, while we were practicing how to teach ChevrYl's Pendulum as a passive test of receptivity—you invite the client to hold a little crystal ball on the end of a chain over a piece of paper that has a circle drawn on it with two lines dissecting it—one vertical, one horizontal. The hypnotist suggests to the client, "please, hold the ball over the middle of the circle, and as you look at the circle, allow your eyes to go back and forth from left to right, back and forth, back and forth." A person who responds well will not only move his eyes back and forth but the ball will start moving back and forth too, as if on its own or through the power of the eye movement. "Now let your eyes go up and down, up and down" "Good, now let your eyes go round and round the circle, round and round." "Now, allow it to go faster and faster, faster and faster." A good hypnotic subject will be able to observe the ball following the path of his eyes. When you ask the subject about the experience they tend to be amazed. "Wow, how did my eyes make the ball move!!! To them, it seems magical, like they have telepathic powers. At that point, you can go right into a hypnosis induction with them, since they are primed and ready.

So as I was saying, while the Chevryl's Pendulum exercise was being demonstrated, my phone vibrated and lit up. That seems pretty magical itself, doesn't it? I looked down and noticed it was my sister. I could check the vm and call her later. Then I saw a text pop up. "Hey u, please call when u have a chance." Uh oh, she's probably having one of her panic attacks. I didn't tell you but I come from a whole family of GAD folk. Hers in the past were very debilitating. I've always worked through mine without anti-depressants and rarely the Valium types. The feeling of her note told me something was wrong. The teacher called a break a little while later, so I left the room, avoiding the steel door to oblivion and called her.

"Hi Sher, I have some bad news."

My heart rate immediately accelerated, "Tell me."

"Aunt Jean had a major stroke. She doesn't recognize anyone and is non-communicative."

"Ohhhh, that's awful."

"She's in the Boca hospital, but it doesn't pay to call, she can't talk or anything. Just so you know where she is."

"Soooo sad . . . ."

This was the same Aunt Jean that tried to soothe me in the Lincoln Tunnel when I was five. I was her favorite niece and she was my favorite aunt. She had two boys, so I kind of became the daughter she wanted.

"And something weird happened. On Saturday, afternoon, Dreya [my cousin] called her and they were chatting. She told Dreya she had to go, because she was going to a show. Dreya asked her who she was going with. She answered, Hanna and Tillie. They're coming to get me shortly."

Hanna and Tillie were her sisters, who had died. I felt a chill go through me.

"What time was that," I asked.

"Around 2, why?"

"Just wondering" I said absently, musing if somehow my anxiety on the massage table and then again today might have been linked to Aunt Jean's potential journey to the other world.

Before my mother died, whenever I got a bladder infection, my mother had one too. I'd call her to say hi, and she'd start complaining about the burning sensation she'd been suffering for days. I had just started the same problem. It happened more times than I can count on my fingers. What the heck was that! Why couldn't I have been "psychically" connected with her being able to whip up an incredible dish in the kitchen instead of a bladder infection?! Phyllis Diller used to have a joke. Her husband got to choose which room she would be good in. It wasn't the kitchen. Me neither.

Actually, I don't think I've had a bladder infection since my mother passed 8 years ago. Hmmmm. So if there is life after death, it must be so nice not to be bothered by bladder and yeast infections. I mean, it's sad that you have to give up on sex, but . . . hopefully there are other joys on the other side that make up for sensual pleasures, ice cream and pizza.

# CHAPTER THIRTY-EIGHT
## "Eclipse of the Heart"

Wow, over 2 weeks since my last post.

Since then, my mother in law had two heart attacks, the second while she was in the ER which was actually a blessing because she was cared for immediately, went into surgery and had a stint implanted. Prognosis is excellent. Phew!

Robin Williams hanged himself.

My niece totaled her car.

My writing coach's wife fell off of her bike and shattered her wrist in 30 places.

My sister in law got a diagnosis of vasculitis which is a fairly serious condition that involves inflammation in the blood vessels and requires steroids,

AND, today and tomorrow our master coaches and coach students are gathering at my home and I realized that I don't have coffee and accouterments for it.

So I'm in the car, outside of Hannaford's our local supermarket, writing instead of being a good hostess and getting what I need. I can just go to Dunkin Donuts and get a few boxes of Jo, right? And they'll give me sides of sweet and white, right? Hope so.

Last night, Glenn and I had our Friday night wind down at Good Karma, our favorite organic restaurant in Exeter, NH. We always get the same things. He gets a huge salad with all kinds of stuff in it and cheesy sauce. It's cheesy because there's no cheese in it. Cheesy name too. I get Asian tempeh over kale. It's soooo good. I'd eat it every day if I could. On the way back, got a call from a prospective coaching student who had signed up for our 10 day test drive, but couldn't do it within the time period because she was a prisoner of ICU. She had just been moved to a regular room and the very first thing she thought of was how to extend her trial period. Isn't it fascinating what becomes most important at various times?

* * *

Spoke with Mom-In-Law. She's still processing what happened to her. Her birthday was last week and she told me she felt very grateful to be alive. Now that she's feeling more confident that she has survived and will continue to improve with little damage if any, she had one regret about her challenging health experience.

"What's that?" I asked.

"Well I could have at least had a near death experience! I was actually disappointed." She laughed. "I thought if anyone would get a peek into what was coming next it would be me. I'm spiritual, accepting and open, but nothing . . . ." She giggled again.

"Awww" I whined in compassionate response. "Right? At least you might have gotten a glimpse into the after-life. Or seen yourself and heard yourself from the ceiling or something, right!?"

"Yeah! But nothing happened. Just pain, more pain and then the pain subsided as they put me under to put the stint in. And then I was back with nothing extra to show for it." She giggled.

"I'm sooooo glad you're back!"

"Yeah, me too."

# CHAPTER THIRTY-NINE
"Relapse?"

I've been sooooo busy that it's been hard to find time to write.

I've been reminded, re-realized that we all have filters through which we see and process the world and our experiences. And sometimes the filters get dirty, further filtering information and sometimes we don't even recognize that it's happening. For instance, I was driving down the street when a ray of light hit the spots on my windshield in such a way that I could barely see out. The glass was covered with water spots or some other coating from the road, trees, weather. I couldn't believe how hard it was to see and how I'd been able to look through it in any light conditions whatsoever with so much covering it. When the bright glare was gone, I once more could see the road and the surrounding vegetation, houses, but as I looked, I realized that all would look a lot different if I cleaned my windshield. Everything was dulled and muted or splotchy. Once it was cleaned, colors were brighter, shapes were clearer, everything was in sharper focus and more readily discernible.

While I was in the crazed phase of attachment with Jill my perceptions of events were different, murkier. It was hard to see the road ahead for the dirty glasses that clouded my vision, thoughts and feelings. I was so concentrated on her that I was missing what was happening in other parts of my world, with other people and events that I could have/might have enjoyed, might have had meaning to me.

Two weeks ago I accidentally sent her an e-book I was in the process of finishing for the academy, "How to Coach Focus." The subject line said, "Latest." I was trying to send it to myself so I could easily open it on my laptop. Her email address is an acronym that starts with my initial and I pushed it without thinking. I've worried that would happen, because whenever I try to send myself something, that address always pops up. And there it finally happened. About half an hour later I got a response,

*Phew!!!!! Thank goodness do you realize how long I have been waiting for this*
*I couldn't resist I hope you're all doing really great!!!!*

So I wrote back . . .

> *"Ha!!!!!*
> *Your name comes up next to mine.*
> *I'll send you the final ;)*
> *Hope all is great."*

I did send her the final a few hours later
She wrote back . . .

> *"Thanks!"*

And then later . . .

> *"PS: it's really good, love how personal it is! Nice work"*

On Saturday, I finished all of my coaching sessions and classes and drove to Whole Foods, which Jill and I always called WTF for short. As I was driving, I got one of those impulses to call her and . . . .

I did.

She doesn't usually answer her phone on Saturdays when she's busy with the kids, but . . . she did.

Me—"Hey its Sharon."

Jill—"Hiiii. I knowwww. How are youuuu?"

Me—"Good [smile in my voice] I guess I wanted to say hi, sending you that e-book."

Jill—"I'm glad you did."

Me—"Your response was really funny . . . I'm still laughing about it."

Jill—"Haaaa. Me too."

We talked for a good 15 minutes. I didn't know what to expect exactly. I think I kind of thought my emotions would be flat after so much time had passed. But it was so natural to talk to her, to laugh with her. I felt joyful.

She told me she thought I didn't want to speak with her. That she had dreams of meeting me where we were always reconciling. That she thought of me all the time and didn't really understand why, why it didn't work.

I told her I thought I did and would be happy to tell her sometime.

"Now is good," she said.

"Uhm, ok . . ." I said a bit hesitantly, a little scared of how this conversation would go. Decided to take as much responsibility as possible for my part . . . .

So, I told her about rapprochement, the stage toddlers go through with their mothers.

Here's an interesting description of this stage of development from the International Encyclopedia of Marriage and Family | 2003:

## Rapprochement

Children begin to realize the limits of their omnipotence and have a new awareness of their separateness and the separateness of the caregiver. Increases in cognition and motor development lead to ambitendency—shadowing and darting away from the caretaker. These behaviors reflect the child's **simultaneous need for autonomy and need for support.** An **increase in aggression is seen in behaviors such as pushing away while whining and clinging.** These behaviors represent the **struggle to reconcile the good and bad aspects of the self and the other, with the need of the** other. Toilet training often begins at this stage, **leading to further struggles with autonomy and control. The verbal no, the developmental milestone of this phase, acts as a metaphor for the issues of autonomy that characterize this stage** (Erikson 1950).

Clinically, the rapprochement period is often cited in conjunction with borderline phenomena, which are characterized by **unstable inner states, unstable relationships, and a fragile sense of self.** In borderline phenomena **there are feelings of loss of support and approval of the other, as well as aggression and anger which arise out of intense feelings of vulnerability and dependency.** The major defenses employed in borderline phenomena *are those of **splitting and projection**. Splitting keeps the "good" and loved aspects of the other separate from the "bad" and hated aspects of the other. **Projection is used to rid oneself of felt unwanted "bad" aspects of the self by attributing those unwanted parts to another**. Internally, because of the lack of integration of the good and bad internal representations of the self and other, individuals with this defensive structure are subject to fluctuating internal states, **feelings of disorganization, and low self-esteem.***

Jill and I got stuck in this struggle with each other, sometimes being the child, sometimes being the parent.

In talking to her about it, I took responsibility for being an over protective mother, not allowing her to feel self-sufficient in her wanderings off, with other friends, with her trip to Virginia. When I told her I was worried when I hadn't heard from her, I triggered her insecurity and made her feel bad about herself/made her question herself. I guessed it made her angry to think I didn't respect or have confidence in her ability to take care of herself, when she was feeling kind of shaky about it herself. I was the over protective, possessive Mommy; she was the toddler, even though she's really an adult doing her best to take care of herself and her kids.

I told her that I realized that I did an instant replay of my Mom, who never wanted me to go off. Instead of supporting her to take care of herself in the best way she knew how to do at the time, I set off an alarm. "Are You OK? I'm worried that I haven't heard from you." I was communicating a sense of concern that she couldn't take care of herself. I mean . . . It was demeaning and disempowering. She was out of town, trying to take care of herself and her kids as best she could and I was sending out an SOS when I didn't hear from her for a day. That's what my mother would have done. "Surala, are you ok? Is there anything the matter? I'm worried about you!!!!" . . . putting dread into my heart. And, that's what I did to Jill.

What I didn't say to her were all of my disappointments in promises broken:

- She gave us a bunch of IOU's for Christmas that she never fulfilled; Tai Body Massage, Yoga lesson, and Paint date.
- But the bigger one, the only one that was really important to me was that I could call on her when I was in trouble and she'd be there. I was totally freaked out at the dentist. I had never used my chits before. The one time I did, was a time she could not fulfill.

Jeremy, my psychoanalytic mentor, tells me that I grossly over-give, overly take care of those I care about to the point of creating princes and princesses who expect more than is reasonable.

But I LOVE to take care of people. It gives me so much pleasure to give to other people. Well, isn't it time to really look at that and figure out how that gets in the way of deep relationships? Do you really always want to be the mother?

I'm not a mother. I wanted to be a mother but it just didn't work out in this life. I have crazy feelings and thoughts about it. Am I not good enough to pass along my DNA? I keep waiting till I get my act together so I don't pass along what my mother did to me. Have I already said this? I felt so betrayed when my sister got pregnant because I thought we had a silent pact NOT to pass along the craziness we grew up with.

She was braver than I was. And even though my sister is a perfectionist, that quality shows up in different areas of her life—the way she makes jewelry or cleans her kitchen. To me, relationships are King. [Or queen?] I do everything I can to make my critical relationships work well.

And here I was totally messing up my relationship with Jill. WTF? [No, Not Whole Foods] How could this be? She meant everything to me and I lost control of my neediness, possessiveness, rational thinking. I'm feeling the tears again, in my chest, my heart. I so wanted to be the best friend she ever had. The most loving Mom, the most understanding soul sister . . . .

But I couldn't. I just couldn't. And what does that mean? Is there meaning here?

Jill is a delicious morsel of chocolate to be savored in the moment. There may not be any left in a minute. Maybe yes? Maybe no!? She has her own struggles of being that happen in tandem and out of tandem with mine. I loved her soooooo deeply. Like I loved my mother who was not capable of loving me in the way I really wanted to be loved. But there was that promise in those so alive eyes and radiant smile . . .

\* \* \*

*An old chief was teaching his grandson about life . . . "A fight is going on inside me," he said to the boy.*

*"It is a terrible fight and it is between two wolves. One is evil—he is anger, envy, sorrow, regret, greed, arrogance, self-pity, guilt, resentment, inferiority, lies, false pride, superiority, self-doubt, and ego. The other is good—he is joy, peace, love, hope, serenity, humility, kindness, benevolence, empathy, generosity, truth, compassion, and faith.*

*"This same fight is going on inside you—and inside every other person, too."*

*The grandson thought about it for a minute and then asked his grandfather,*

*"Which wolf will win?"*

*The old chief simply replied,*

*"The one you feed."*

When will I stop being hungry for Jill . . .

# CHAPTER FORTY
"Laksmi—Goddess Mother of Mine"


A few years ago, my spiritual Swami took me on a meditative journey where I was invited to go between lives. He asked me to close my eyes and drift . . . . To drift to a time way back, Back, back, back. Years passing before my eyes and ears and senses until it was a time before I was born . . . . He invited me to explore the space, the moment I found before I was born. I was in a beautiful tropical garden full of color, sounds and scents. And the temperature was just right. I walked through the lush vegetation, feeling the moisture in the air, hearing the sounds of birds and wild life nearby, smelling interesting scents of indigenous flowers and plants and, and, what is that? Something I couldn't define.

I created my own path through the trees and vines and found myself in a clearing that was just . . .

beautiful, vibrant, and emotionally satisfying, I can't even describe it well. I see a BEAUTIFUL woman with long, straight, shiny black hair sitting on an ornate throne of bamboo, I think. She smiles broadly and motions for me to approach. Lithe, women in some kind of loose fitting diaphanous pantaloons and gauzy tops with flowing long, dark hair are slowly waving giant fronds in her direction. Air conditioning? Really? OK, let's see what happens. I approach. She looks at me with the most inviting smile and I hear in my mind at first, like a whisper. daaauuughhhter. Then with an eagerness to her tone and lightness in her pitch, DAUGHTER!? . . . Daughter!?

Mother? I think tentatively. Wha!? This is a majestic woman, my mother was tiny and round. But I find myself compelled and I approach closer and closer, feeling my chest swell with . . . love?

'Please,' she smiles and motions me forward.

I go to her like a toddler, waddling, feeling my awkward footing as I approach. As I get within 2 feet of her, she reaches down and picks me up as if I'm tiny and draws me to her chest. I feel . . . joy, fulfillment, amazement, delight, silliness, laughter, sadness, tears of relief as she hugs me to her firm, full breasts. And as she does, a myriad of images fill and swirl through my consciousness. I see myself in ballet class, running in the woods, pushing my fingers into clay and forming figures, in math class raising my hand, in chemistry

289

running my hand over the periodical chart and mysteriously changing the symbols, in a gathering of women toning and drumming, in an athletic class picking up kettle bells, at an archeological dig with a quizzical look on my face, at a funeral crying and saying goodbye, in a convertible with my hair whipping my face as I drive up a mountain road.

In my mind's ear, I hear, "objects may be closer than they appear" and I pause and look up into her ecstatic face. "Yes," beloved, "yes", She glows at me. She's smiling so intensely that I think her lips can actually meet her ears! Is that possible, my rational mind inquires trying to make sense of what I'm experiencing? She's not Jack Nicolson as the Riddler. Thank God! But what is this? Who is she? Who am I?

I decide to let go of my rational deliberations. I recognize something in her that feels very familiar. She's different but the same. We share something so vital and exciting that I can hardly hold the feeling. I can't hold it, it's a wave of joy that connects my heart with hers a gently humming rose pink glow that expands from our connection and radiates out and out and out slowly at first but then growing faster to encompass all around us. Her smile ignites mine and I feel peace and jubilation at the same time. I feel in love with life, with her, with myself, with everything around me and not around me.

This is beyond exciting. So ecstatic! Is this what a profound religious/spiritual experience feels like? The pink gold tinged glow that now encompasses everything begins to settle down. The hum is quieting. I'm back in the recliner chair gently opening my eyes. Wow . . . What was that?

He nods at me, eyes at half mast.

I stay with my sweet feelings of serene inspiration. I had been sooooo angry at my birth mother for so many years that allowing myself to have this ideal mother in this reverie was a revelation. It made me realize that I was finally beginning to truly love myself and give to myself what I needed. I didn't have to wait for my mother to take care of me, I could take care of myself. Cleansing, joyful tears washed the windshield of my mind allowing me to see the radiance that illuminated everything around me. Just for a very intense moment, I could see details in the room that I had been missing, recall overtures of friendship from others I had unintentionally dismissed, feel the soft gust of cool air that whispered gently in my ear as it wisped my hair from my face, smell the scent of . . . bergamot?

I suddenly wake from my reverie. Why am I thinking bergamot? I don't even know what bergamot is and don't know if I would recognize it if I did. Back in Beta brain wave, I jump to the internet to see what it is and if there's any symbolism attached to it.

Hmmmm. Let's see, I think to myself hoping for some amazing metaphysical revelation. Oh, man TDW is gazing at my laptop from over my right shoulder.

Looking like that 1500 year old Matthew—the long black haired, white faced vampire with a conscience, who wears a cross and is not affected by sunlight, nor does he sparkle—in Deborah Harkness's A Discovery of Witches trilogy. Was that the cool breeze I felt!?

"Would you please step back a little!" I think at him. He raises his hands palms open in acquiescence and steps back a bit.

"Lets' see," I muse out loud, as I sort through the many references.

> *During citrus season in France, if you're lucky, you'll run across something called a **bergamot**. They're not brilliant yellow like regular lemons, but a sort of orangey color, and when split open, they're quite juicy and the flavor is much sweeter than regular lemons. In fact, they often call them citrons doux, which translates to "sweet lemons."*

"Oh, yes," TDW interjects from his perch on the desk behind me. We used to use them in teas; very nice flavor, not too tart.

"Shhhhh . . . I'm trying to concentrate," I hiss at him.

> *Bergamot is very useful for problems with the digestive system, such as flatulence, abdominal cramps, and gastro-enteritis.*

"Heh-heh-heh," he snickers. "Well that would be good for this family, especially the dog!"

"OMG! Even spirits or, or . . . whatever you are . . . have potty humor! Must be a male thing!!" I say with irritation.

*It's used for agitation, anxiety, and insomnia. It's also good for cuts and wounds, dermatitis, greasy skin and psoriasis.*

"Well there's one for you, Mr. Greasy!" I snipe at him.

"Reeeaaalllly!?" he looked at me with one eyebrow raised. "Have you looked at my flawless skin recently?"

"Actually . . . ? I try to look at you as little as possible!?" Ugh, I'll never be able to compete with him in sarcasm. Can't believe I got seduced into a nasty repartee!!!

*Please note, that Bergamot is the MOST photo-sensitive of all the citrus oils, so please wait 12-24 hours after using it, to go Sun Bathing or using a sun bed.*

"Wait, if you're a vampire, what are you doing in the sunlight?"

"I never said I was a vampire. You read far too many goofy novels, you know"

I kept searching and reading.

> *Bergamot oil is considered sedative and healing and used for stress related problems, depression and anxiety.*

"Now finally that's what you need!" He said with a little burst of excitement in his usually mocking tone. "Maybe I could go rest for a while instead of having to be so watchful over you."

"No one asked you to watch over me!" Arrrgh . . . . He's sooooo . . . annoying.

"Didn't they? Are you so sure of that?"

I dismiss him and return to my screen.

> *"Increases physical and magical energy and increases the flow of money into your life. It can also help to ensure that you spend wisely and take advantage of offers to earn more."*

Simultaneously we both say, "INTERESTING!!!"

I turn my head slowly and look at him quizzically, "Lakshmi sent you?"

"Not sure . . . I thought it was the dude on the mountain with the golden wings, but . . . hmmmm, I don't really believe in all of that mumbo jumbo, you know . . ."

"Whaaaah . . . !? Uhm, waaaaah . . . !?" I was speechless. He doesn't believe in . . . OK, this is just too weird.

I thought of Lakshmi because she is the Hindi Goddess of abundance—often associated with financial prosperity, but to me she is the embodiment of goodness, graciousness, the all perfect mother, the woman I met between lives.

I have statues of Lakshmi in my home and office as a reminder of her generous gifts of love and the wealth of all good things. She helps me grow in a grounded garden of possibilities. People always comment on the spaces where she lives with us as enchanting, supposedly complementing our décor, but I know it is Lakshmi's benevolent blessings they feel. I'm grateful for having met her between lives.

"And what about yours truly . . . ?" He asks with a smirk. "Aren't you grateful for finally meeting me too?"

"Uhm . . . ." I wanted to say No, but actually I WAS intrigued by my personal mystery man or monster or whatever he was. "I am certainly curious about you and you have gotten me out of a couple of bad moments, which I am grateful for . . . but I still don't understand why you hang around and what you are and who you are and why me, and . . . ."

"Shhh, shhh, shhhhhh," He quieted me. "All in good time . . . . Sorry for teasing you so much. Just makes my existence a bit more fun, but I know I shouldn't bother you. But you get so testy and fired up that it makes me laugh. You're just so tempting to annoy."

My face colored as anger filled my chest and arms. He was definitely cruising.

"Oooops, there, I just did it again, didn't I! Sorry. I'll try to behave." He lowered his head and cast down his eyes.

"Oh quit the fake humility. Just tell me why you are here."

"I'm not sure quite frankly. But I know we have a task or two . . . or three . . . or four. Not quite sure. They send me. I go."

"They . . . ?"

"Ooops, again . . . sorry . . . . This will all make sense in the end. But for now, you seem fine, I'm off"

And then he was . . . off the edge of the desk, off into thin air. Not there.

I blinked and opened my eyes and took in a breath. I'm just never quite sure if he's a day dream, hypnotic trance element or a psychotic delusion, or . . . some kind of shape shifter, super natural being? Really?! Well, he's definitely interesting in any case, fig newton or not.

*TDW speaks:* If you're interested in getting to know TDW a little more, he has started his own blog.

Wouldn't you know!! He's so full of himself. You can access it here: www.GetLostGirlfriend.com

I wrote a story in Kiddy Lit for 5-8 year olds when I was 20. We had to write the copy, illustrate it and bind it. I thought it was a spin on what happened with me and a friend when I was 15. I had a revelation about it a few days ago in relation to my Jill travails now so many years later. It was called Forever Friends.

In Kiddy Lit, we were taught to put an illustration on the left page and a few short lines on the right. It's interesting because it reflects what I learned in creating ads. Visual goes on left for best uptake and copy on right. So that's what I did: simple illustrations on left and short copy on right. I tried finding the book that was made with art paper and bound with dental floss but alas it's either in hiding or gone.

The story went something like this. It started out . . .

Julie Ann and Lisa were forever friends. Every morning at 7am, Julie Ann kissed her baby sister on her forehead, picked up her Happy Days lunch box with a sandwich on white bread, a couple of cheese balls, a red Delicious apple and hopefully a Twinkie, said good bye to her Mom and walked across the street to Lisa's house.

She'd lift the giant door knocker and let it drop— even though she could have wrung the bell, the door knocker was more fun—and then wait until Mrs.

Parker came to the door. "Lisa will be right out, Julie Ann," Mrs. Parker smiled at her.

Julie Ann smiled back and waited on the stoop for Lisa to appear.

The two walked arm and arm all the way to school talking about this and that and giggling about everything.

They sat together at lunch, played together at recess. And every day at 3:00 sharp they left school together and walked home arm in arm, talking about this and that and giggling about everything.

Julie Ann and Lisa were Forever Friends . . . Until . . . SHE moved in.

That girl with the shiny gold pigtails, big blue eyes . . . . And Raggedy Ann Freckles on her face

When Julie Ann knocked on Lisa's door, Mrs. Parker said, "Oh my dear. Lisa has already left. She must be a block or two up with that sweet new girl Rachel."

Julie Ann's mouth dropped in shock. Lisa left?

Julie Ann thanked Mrs. Parker, turned and slowly started walking to school all by herself. That day was a very sad day.

Julie Ann ate lunch all by herself. Lisa was nowhere to be found. Julie Ann went to recess all by herself and sat on a swing all alone. She looked around for Lisa at the end of the day, but no Lisa. Julie Ann was so sad. She walked home all by herself and went right to her room when she got home and didn't come out till her mother called her for dinner.

I can't remember exactly how I resolved the story— why did Lisa leave without waiting for Julie Ann? What were they doing without her? What made them finally decide to include her? But I do remember the last couple of pages. Lisa and Rachel came, calling for Julie Ann, and all three go off to school together. The last page declared, "Three forever friends were better than two".

Honestly, I never believed that . . . . In the illustration—that I drew—Lisa and the new girl have their free arms around each other, while Julie Ann has her arm on Lisa's shoulder with a somewhat annoyed look on her face even though she's smiling. I'm actually a little surprised that no one called me on it. Julie Ann looked like the 5th wheel. I thought I SHOULD think, feel, that there could be three forever friends, that it was politically correct, but I've never been one to want to be part of any triangle. So it wasn't a satisfying ending to the story.

AND, you know how I've been saying that the sense of abandonment by Jill has been a reflection of the difficult relationship with my mother? When I thought about the Forever Friends book, I had a major aha that the betrayal had to do with the birth of my sister! I was the only little girl and then my sister was born. I felt displaced, but guilty. I was supposed to love my sister. I mean, I had prayed for her for a whole year. She was born two days after my birthday.

Little baby, cute as a button. Like the old Talking Heads song "cute, cute as a button. Don't you wanna make him stay up late . . ." She was sooo cute.

But, Little sister got my bed, my favorite old clothes—including my beautiful red Mexican jacket that I loved when I was 2, my hand painted dresser and the attention of both of my parents. She was the apple of Daddy's eye. Whatever she did was adorable. Whatever I did . . . well what did I do? Who knows? No one noticed. I just faded into the background with the exception of those moments when I got in trouble being "bad."

How I dealt with it was to become my sister's mother. I think I actually believed that she came to life out of my wish for her to exist and my prayers. She was like my little doll. Even though I was only 5 I quickly learned how to take care of her, feed her, help bathe her, assist in diapering, entertain her. As she grew, I taught her how to walk, talk. I played with her, pushed her on the swing set that we got for her [not for me, for her.] I took her to school and walked her home. I helped her with her homework. We shared a room. When she had scary dreams I talked her down. I protected her from our big scary brothers, from bullies in school.

And, she really loved me. Throughout my life she's been the one person who I've always known has loved me no matter what . . . even if she usurped my place of being the baby in the family.

When things went down with Jill for the second time and I felt so alone, my sister was there to listen and support. She has been a true friend.

I've been thinking that I treated Jill the way I did my baby sister. At first, the connection was magical, like finding the goddess Lakshmi in my reverie—all giving, all accepting, fulfilling all my needs as the most intuitive of mothers, knowing what I wanted and needed as I did. But then, when we ran into a snag— her weekend with her other best friend—we got back together by my swallowing my needs and becoming the sister to her that I was to my baby sister. I stifled my feelings of rejection and took on the role of caregiver.

That worked out with my sister, because she really was a baby and I was the elder for a long time, guiding and teaching. It's only recently after many years become more of an equal relationship, although once the big sister, always the big sister.

But with Jill, it was a defensive maneuver that was driven by fear and then desperation. I had to take care of her and suppress my feelings for fear of her leaving again. And, then of course, she did.

Things can get so convoluted and complex in relationships.

SHARON LIVINGSTON, Ph. D.

Have you ever seen the book "Knots" by psychiatrist R D Laing?

He reminds me how I've at times twisted myself into a pretzel to escape from feeling abandoned, devastated, loss of self-esteem. Check out this one, an excerpt from his book . . .

> There must be something the matter with him
> Because he would not be acting as he does
> Unless there was
> Therefore he is acting as he is
> Because there is something the matter with him
> He does not think there is anything the matter with him
> Because one of the things that is
> The matter with him is that he does not think that there is anything
> The matter with him
> Therefore
> We have to help him realize that,
> The fact that he does not think there is anything
> The matter with him
> Is one of the things that is
> The matter with him
> There is something the matter with him
> Because he thinks
> There must be something the matter with us
> For trying to help him to see

That there must be something the matter with
him
To think that there is something the matter with
us
For trying to help him to see that
We are helping him
To see that
We are not persecuting him
By helping him
To see we are not persecuting him
By helping him
To see that
He is refusing to see
That there is something the matter with him
For not seeing there is something the matter with
him
For not being grateful to us
For at least trying to help him
To see that there is something the matter with
him
For not seeing that there must be something the
matter with him
For not seeing that there must be something the
matter with him
For not seeing that there is something the matter
with him
For not seeing that there is something the matter
with him

SHARON LIVINGSTON, Ph. D.

For not being grateful
That we never tried to make him

Feel grateful."Reeaaaaaally?" TDW is back. He's draped over the chair that Stewie usually occupies and is staring at my computer monitor. "That's very weird indeed. What's the problem with that chap Laing? Are his synapses misfiring?"

I'm pacing in the small space behind my stability ball.

"I want to fire you!" I snap.

"My dear . . . . This discombobulating of phraseology would snarl any protective being to come to your immediate aid."

"Stop! Everything is fine," I say. "Just trying to understand . . . everything . . . ." I flop down on my ball.

"Why?" He pushes himself up from the chair and slowly approaches me holding my gaze, intently but gently. I see caring in his face rather than poking fun at me. It seems like he's really trying to understand . . . me. He stops a couple of feet away from me, drops to an easy crouch and continues to hold a steady calm gaze.

"I . . . don't know exactly," I stammer, a little shy in light of his fixed attention.

I feel tears pushing behind my eyes and my face warming.

"What?" He asks gently.

"I, I've always wanted someone's complete attention and here I seem to have it from . . . you and, and, yet, it makes me uncomfortable." My eyes cast down shyly.

"From me . . . ?!" He says softly, sounding incredulous. "TDW? Really? I'm totally harmless . . . to you. You must know that by now."

"You know, I kind of do."

"I've never actually been afraid of you, more amazed and curious and sometimes annoyed, but not afraid. I think I know you can't or wouldn't harm me. You've never even said 'Boo' or tried to shock me."

"Well you've always had a very strong startle response . . ." he muses, "as I recall, even when you were in the womb, you would start when your big brother approached your mother . . ."

"Victor? That big brother . . . ?"

"Yes"

"Well he's the one that made me roll out of bed and fracture my collar bone when I was two!" I sputter indignantly.

He takes my chin in his hand and gently draws my face back to looking into his eyes. "Sorry, I didn't mean to upset you. Yes, you're right. He was a bit of a devil that one; tortured soul, really. But he'll get another chance." Soft eyes, lips slightly curved upwards.

Oh my God, is he going to kiss me?!

"No, dear heart," he chokes a little and guffaws. "We are way beyond any of those earthly shenanigans."

"But you are here and now and alive and real, aren't you?"

"I AM here"

"And you have such an interesting life, don't you. You have that special ability of looking and listening and seeing things others often glaze over or miss, right here, right now in everyday occurrences. You said it yourself; you are gifted with intensity, correct?"

"Well, yes. But I'm only beginning to understand that as a gift. It's been a problem in the past because it would spur me to impulsively react and get myself in trouble and . . . ."

"Shhhh. It's OK. We're figuring it alllll out, little one."

I pull back, uncomfortable with the endearment. "Why, do you keep calling me, 'little one'?!"

He retreats to his mocking mode. "Oh, you're sooooo big, aren't you?!" He laughs at me, but I can still see softness in his eyes.

TDW straightens up and steps back, cocks his head to his right shoulder as if he's listening to someone, some thing . . . .

"Gotta go, girl. I'll see you . . . when I see you. You're good for now I see."

He flashes me a smile and in a non-flash, as if nothing had happened, as if he was never there, he was not there.

Hmmmmm. This Lesson Seven—Life is an Adventure—has been a longer one than I expected. But how apropos, right? I intend to live a very long and meaningful life, filled with interesting people, problems and solutions, inquiry, observations, scientific evidence, hypotheses and musings from my intellect, heart, soul, intuition, instincts and creative mind.

Mind!? What is mind? Wikipedia?

> *A mind is the set of cognitive faculties that enables consciousness, perception, thinking, judgement, and memory—a characteristic of humans, but which also may apply to other life forms.[3][4]*
>
> *A lengthy tradition of inquiries in philosophy, religion, psychology and cognitive science has sought to develop an understanding of what a mind is and what its distinguishing properties are. The main question regarding the nature of mind is its relation to the physical brain and nervous system—a question which is often framed as the Mind-body problem, which considers whether mind is somehow separate from physical existence (dualism and idealism[5]), deriving from and/or reducible to physical phenomena such as neuronal activity (physicalism), or whether the mind is*

*identical with the brain or some activity of the brain.[6] Another question concerns which types of beings are capable of having minds, for example whether mind is exclusive to humans, possessed also by some or all animals, by all living things, or whether mind can also be a property of some types of man-made machines.*

*Whatever its relation to the physical body it is generally agreed that mind is that which enables a being to have subjective awareness and intentionality towards their environment, to perceive and respond to stimuli with some kind of agency, and to have consciousness, including thinking and feeling . . . Some of the earliest recorded speculations linked mind (sometimes described as identical with soul or spirit) to theories concerning both life after death, and cosmological and natural order, for example in the doctrines of Zoroaster, the Buddha, Plato, Aristotle, and other ancient Greek, Indian and, later, Islamic and medieval European philosophers.*

Ohhh. VERY complex!!! That's a can of worms for another fisherman or woman.

I'm about to bring this part of the story to temporary closure.

I say temporary, because I realize in writing down my thoughts and feelings over the past 6 months, I've discovered that I LOVE to write, and . . . if you would have me . . . I would be honored and delighted to share more of my musings with you.

I received a note from Jill earlier this week. It was a simple question about supplements. Around here I'm kind of known as the vitamin and supplement queen. If you saw the shelves in my laundry room and stash in my basement you'd think I was running my own store.

She shot over a request for something on "immunity", hers seemed to be run down. So I asked her a couple of questions. It went like this.

Jill: Hi there,

Hope you had a great weekend I had a quick question for you if you don't mind. If you had to recommend one supplement to boost immunity what would it be? I have a hard time from September to March and I can already feel myself changing I need a boost? Thank you so much I just wasn't sure if you have tried something that worked, there are so many out there.

Me: Hey,

I'm going to see Dr. Morrison today. I can ask him.

Glenn hasn't gotten ANY colds since he eats mushrooms, onions and berries everyday BTW. Pretty impressive!

But Doc Dale will have a supp recommendation I'm sure.

Jill: Okay thanks. You don't have to do that. It's okay. Maybe I will just start eating mushrooms, onions and berries :D. Thanks again!

Me: My pleasure; would be great to hear :)

Jill: Okay, great. Thank you, I appreciate it. I just wasn't sure if there was one that you guys were already using. Thanks so much!!

Me: Three recs:

Biggest, Cut out sugar

Fish oil for general immunity

Lysine for cold sores

Hope that helps

And hope little one feels better.

Jill: Thanks, makes sense. Thanks for asking.

And that was that.

So why was I sharing such an emotion free communication?

It's because I realized that the addictive quality of my relationship with Jill seems to be healed. I mean the question still remains, can I hang out around chocolate without over indulging. I'm not sure, but I haven't had sugar in a long time and am fine without it.

And . . . I dunno . . . . And how interesting is this kind of communication? Is this what I want in a friendship? Casual acquaintance . . . ? Maybe . . . ? Maybe not . . . .

I do know that even though there are those who say they prefer a peaceful, calm life without drama, I know that I like my intensity. Does that make me bi-polar? Manic? I love living in high definition and vibrant hues at moments while simultaneously, taking in the scents and sounds and subtleties of experience.

That's probably why I'm so susceptible to addictive substances—be they sweets or charismatic people. I like the engagement, the stimulation, and the tug on my heart.

When it comes down to it, I love to feel . . . deeply.

And when I think about the resolve with Jill, in the end, NOTHING HAPPENED!

There's a children's book called The Camel Who Took a Walk. The resolve is that nothing happened. It's just a story of taking a walk and seeing what you see and hearing what you hear and feeling what you feel.

To me, the excitement in life is the journey and my experiences along the way. I guess it doesn't really matter how it turns out in the end. Because, while we're alive and living, there really is no end!

* * *

I picture myself getting in my Honda Accord, Stewie riding side-saddle on his sheepskin seat cover. The sedan is magically transformed into a sleek red Ferrari with the top down. I'm wearing a long lightweight scarf around my head to protect my hair from tangling and giant black sunglasses, Stewie is wearing a pair of custom shades for Shih Tzu's. We get on the nearest highway and start to drive. I feel a touch on my shoulder and realize its TDW. He thinks at me, "Let's go! On to the next adventure . . . ." I smile and drive . . .

> Life is a highway; I wanna ride it
> All night long.
> If you're going my way, I wanna drive it
> All night long.

Rascal Flatts—Life Is A Highway Lyrics | MetroLyrics

## WOULD YOU LIKE TO LEARN HOW TO BECOME YOUR OWN BEST FRIEND?

Go to www.howtobeyourownbestfriend.com for some things I discovered that you might consider, too, for being good to yourself.

# ACKNOWLEDGMENTS

Some events in life may seem so devastating that we feel as if we're being destroyed, down to our core. At those moments, the impact on our self esteem is so powerful, so irrevocable, that we can't even look in the mirror. But, the truth is we have a choice. We can reframe painful experiences into opportunities. We can choose to grow from them. I had such an experience with a talented, brilliant woman who I thought was my best friend. At first I was so hurt that I could hardly function. After ranting and raving inside myself, talking it out with my husband and multiple "therapists," I started to heal, repair, regain my sense of humor, explore anew, grow and discover myself all over again.

Writing a book is not a solitary event. It requires help, guidance, support, feedback and inspiration from a number of people. Without the help of many special people who I can't thank enough, this book could not have come to life and been so cathartic and transformational for me.

To my new found dearest friend, exuberant cheerleader and super advocate, Esther Gendelman. How lucky am I that Jill left so I had the space to reflect and grow and recognize you when you meandered into my life. I feel so blessed to have a true friend who is with me through thick and thin, willing to ride the waves and storms of life, to live, laugh, love [as the plaque over my sink says] AND who is willing to trust and depend on me when she navigates her own murky waters as well as flying high through clear skies. I love my Esther.

Penni Hauck—my sister who let me complain and complain and cry and 'yamagoash' about it all. You know me longer than any other person and continued to love me and play with me, no matter what. I'm so grateful for you.

Doug Lipman—my amazing story telling coach and new found friend, who lit my creative writing flame and encouraged me to share my voice, even when I sometimes couldn't hear it myself.

John Chancellor—my rock and constant firm but gentle inspirer who saw me emerging in my life and writing competencies and cheered me on no matter what.

Yoav Ezer—my brother from another mother who teaches me how to get the word out and publish and laughs with me at all the right moments.

My readers, fellow coaches and dear friends who appreciated my stories and spurred me on Renee Asmar, Jayne Logan, Helen Thorgalsen, Jen May, Catherine Miller.

Steve Harrison and Jack Canfield for appearing in my life at just the right moment to almost magically springboard me into another dimension of my career, purpose and mission.

And, finally but most importantly to my life partner, husband, playmate, my mommy, my daddy and my dog, Glenn Livingston. You held me and fortified me with tenderness and caring, intriguing questions to help me learn and your ever present humor to joke me out of my darkest self flagellating moments. You reminded me I was lovable when I felt so abandoned. You even played friend-therapist to help me take a different perspective and see myself in a new life.

And lastly to "Jill" who will probably never see this. Thank you for helping me look at a broken part of myself and forcing me to have the courage to look in the mirror and see the real me.

## ABOUT THE AUTHOR
### Sharon Livingston, Ph.D.

For over 25 years Dr. Sharon Livingston, founder and president of The Livingston Group for Emotional Marketing, has been one of the most prominent leaders in the field of motivational research and Insight Mining.

Dr. Livingston is President of ICCA—The international Coach Certification Alliance, CoachCertiicationAlliance.com, an organization dedicated to professional personal coach training excellence.

She has been a mentor for HBA—the Healthcare Business Women's Association for almost 10 years.

Sharon and her beloved husband and brilliant business partner Dr. Glenn Livingston

co-authored a large scale 5 year study on body language of attraction and dating. The results were used to write a successful e-book, "How to Use Body Language" which sold 37,000 copies.

Dr. Livingston holds a Ph.D. in Psychology, is an NGH [National Guild of Hypnotists] Hypnosis Trainer, an NLP practitioner and has had extensive training in creative ideation procedures, group dynamics, applied psychological techniques, and projective methods. Her dissertation proved that a photo-sort successfully predicted scores on the Myers Brigg Personality Inventory.

She was a finalist for the 2008 Enterprising Woman of the Year award, and in June of 2015 was voted an Outstanding Woman of the year by the New England Family Business Association.

Sharon and Glenn live in NH with their adorable dog children Stewie and Jeremy. She enjoys painting, hiking, helping others and making people laugh. Glenn and Sharon cultivate a loving, extended "family" of inspired coaches globally. This passionate community lights up the hearts of all those that have the privilege to work with them.

Go to www.GetLostGirlfriend.com to learn about her other books and the programs she offers.

Made in the USA
Middletown, DE
07 March 2016